A Medical Gentleman:
JAMES J. WARING M.D.

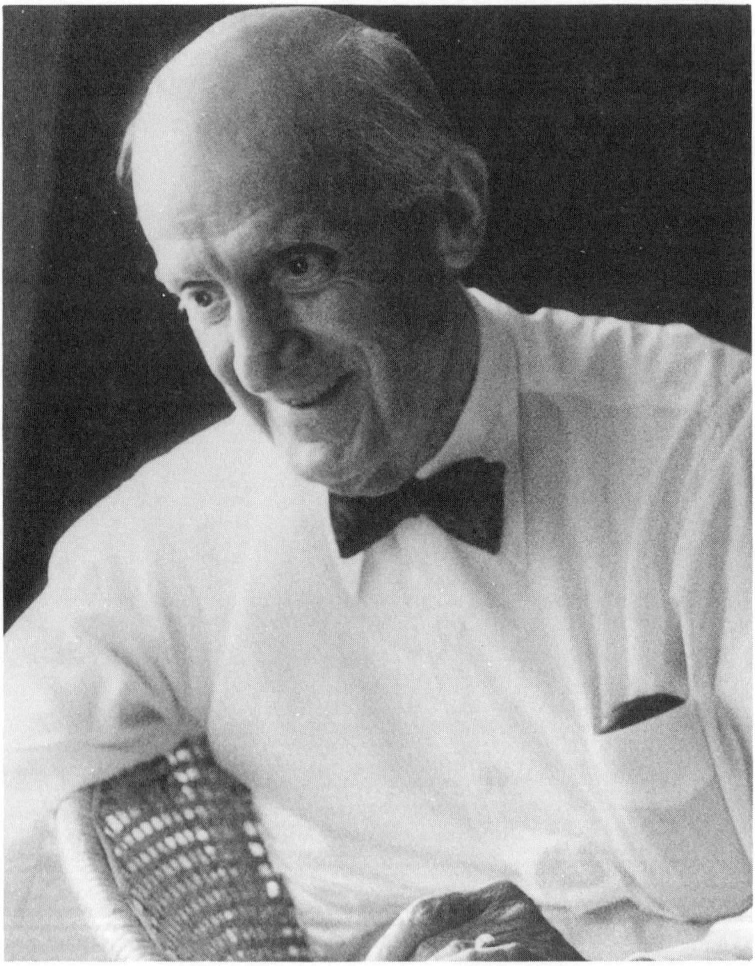

A Medical Gentleman: JAMES J. WARING M.D.

by Patricia Paton

Colorado Historical Society 1993

This publication was made possible in part by a grant from the Colorado Endowment for the Humanities

Library of Congress Cataloging-in-Publication Data

Paton, Patricia, 1927–
A medical gentleman : James J. Waring, M.D. / by Patricia Paton
p. cm.
Includes bibliographical references and index.
ISBN 0-942576-33-0 (pbk.). — ISBN 0-942576-02-0 (hardcover)
1. Waring, James J. 1883–1962. 2. Physicians—Colorado—Biography. 3. Tuberculosis—Treatment—History. I. Title
[DNLM: 1. Waring, James J. 1883–1962. 2. Physicians—biography. 3. Tuberculosis—history. WZ 100 W276P 1993]
R154.W227P38 1993
610'.92—dc20
[B]
DNLM/DLC
for Library of Congress 93-23589

Contents

Acknowledgments

Credit for the inception of this biography goes to Anne Waring Maer and Ruth Waring Halpenny, daughters of James J. Waring. Writing about someone one does not know might have been formidable were it not for James Waring's cooperative family. Anne Waring Maer, living in the same city as I, bore the major share of my questioning and gave valuable editorial assistance throughout many versions of the manuscript. Ruth Waring Halpenny of Riverside, California, and I had one long meeting, then corresponded concerning early versions of the manuscript. I thank them for not trying to shape or censor this biography of their father; they allowed me to make my own assessment and interpretation. I was given free range of a treasure of family correspondence, among them James Waring's letters to family and friends and his mother's letters to her two sons. Thanks go to Dr. William Waring, Dr. Antonio Waring's son and Jane B. Aron Professor of Pediatrics at Tulane School of Medicine, for making many of these letters available. Dr. Francis Trudeau gave permission to publish letters from his grandfather, Dr. Edward L. Trudeau, to Dr. Waring. Mrs. Gail LaForge gave permission to publish a letter from her father, Dr. Herbert M. Evans.

Of special help was a thirty-one-page biography by Dr. Paul N. Anderson, written when he was a student, for presentation to a Waring Society symposium in 1963. Dr. Anderson corresponded with many of Dr. Waring's colleagues, most of whom are now gone.

The book—some of the early chapters, in particular—benefited from the considerable groundwork laid by writer Mary Cable; thanks go to her for her many contributions.

Edward D. White III, a grandson of James Waring, gave me two large boxes of files, on loan from the Colorado Historical Society, which told of Dr. Waring's paper on pneumothorax. Ted and his father, Edward D. White Jr., also read the manuscript and offered suggestions.

Dr. Henry Toll Jr., a family friend, provided information about James Waring, book collector; the Webb-Waring Lung Institute; and other matters. Pauline Riedeburg Plesset, another family friend, provided penetrating observations about Jim and Ruth Waring. Houstoun Waring told humorous family tales. Dr. John Lunt told about his father's long friendship with Dr. Waring. Jeanne Erskine and Mary Filley told of their friendship with Ruth Porter Waring, and they and Louise Graber gave details about the musical group to which they all belong.

Professional associates of Dr. Waring gave me valuable assistance. Dr. Roger Mitchell patiently gave advice on medical details. (In 1980 he received the prestigious Trudeau Medal of the National Tuberculosis Association, as had Dr. Waring before him.) Dr. David Talmage offered suggestions, and Alfred Crowle, Ph.D., and M. Laurance Morse, Ph.D., reviewed selected scientific details, as did John E. Repine, M.D., director of the Webb-Waring Lung Institute, and Joe M. McCord, Ph.D., of the institute. Drs. Ben Eiseman and Roger Wotkyns told about the Waring Society.

Henry Swan II, M.D., told about postwar planning at the University of Colorado School of Medicine and about fishing with Dr. Waring. E. Stewart Taylor, M.D., shed further light on various views of James Waring. J. Cuthbert Owens, M.D., told about Dr. Waring's physical condition in his later years. Dr. George Wright was a valuable source of information on industrial medicine. Jean Blount gets credit for the book's title.

Thanks go also to all those with whom I corresponded, including Drs. S. G. Scadding and W. H. Helm, who wrote with clear recall of Dr. Waring's visit to Britain three and a half decades before. Among those who were helpful, whether through an interview in person or by telephone, or correspondence, are: Alice Bishop-Ring, M.D.; Robert Bosworth, M.D.; George Bower, M.D.; Robert K. Brown, M.D.; Winona Campbell, M.D.; Kenneth Caughey; Robert Chapman, M.D.; Cornelia (Mrs. Frank) Church; J. Philip Clarke, M.D.; William Condon, M.D.; George Curfman, M.D.; John Denst, M.D.; John Durrance, M.D.; Elaine Ellis; Charles Freed, M.D.; Stanley Friesen, M.D., Ph.D.; William Gambill, Ph.D.; Mitten Gates (Mrs. Harry); Ruth Gorham; Paul Halley; Lucile Harrington; Mason Howard, M.D.; Robert Hudson, M.D.; Herbert Hultgren, M.D.; Harriot Hunter, M.D. (Mrs. Robert Jardine); Walter Huttner, M.D.; Mabel Ingram (Mrs. Fred); Robert Jardine, M.D.; Dalton Jenkins, M.D.; Melvin Johnson, M. D.; Mary Barkalow (Mrs. Robert) Joyce; Wallace Livingston, M.D.; Lula Lubchenco, M.D.; Michael Lubchenco, M.D.; Ranald MacDonald; William Maniatis, M.D.; Jane McGilvray; Gordon Meiklejohn, M.D.; Mason Morfit, M.D.; Naomi Minner Morris, M.D.; George Ogura, M.D.; Thomas Petty, M.D.; Herbert Rothenberg, M.D.; Shimpei Sakaguchi, M.D.; Jonas Schreider, M.D.; Charley Smyth, M.D.; Stuart Schneck, M.D.; James Swallow, M.D.; William Waring, M.D.; Robert Weiner, M.D.; and Seymour Wheelock, M.D.

Patricia Nelson, who was head of Special Collections and is now associate director of Denison Memorial Medical Library of the University of Colorado, and Abby Johnson enabled me to utilize books and papers in the secured area of the Waring Room. Mary DeMund of the Denver Medical Society Library and Cathy Canzonetta of the University of Colorado School of Medicine's Alumni Office were not fazed by my many questions. Librarians at the Colorado Historical Society assisted me in my quest, as did those of the Western History Department and branches of the Denver Public Library. Yale University's alumni office was helpful, as was that of the Lawrenceville School and of the Johns Hopkins School of Medicine; archivists at Yale and Hopkins helped, too. Bernice Petersen and librarians Solange Gignac and Ellen Mackey provided details on the Denver Botanic Gardens. The late Peter Olch, M.D., medical historian, helped trace a medical school's history. Assistance came from archivists of the University of California, San Francisco, and the Georgia Historical Society, Savannah.

Charles Houston, M.D., professor emeritus of the University of Vermont, was kind enough to edit selected chapters. Mark S. Foster, chairman of the History Department at the University of Colorado at Denver, was helpful in paring down the oversized manuscript, and Marilyn Amer of the English Department of that institution, and Tim McGovern also read various versions and offered suggestions. Lastly, Bruce Paton, my physician husband, was a great support, answering medical questions, reading the manuscript, solving word processor problems and living with the ups and downs of producing a book.

The Colorado Historical Society deserves special thanks for its support of this project in its later stages. Thanks also go to James C. Pierce and Maggie Coval of the Colorado Endowment for the Humanities for help in securing a generous grant to assist in the the publication of this book..

There are many more people who have helped, but space limitations prevent mentioning them by name. My thanks to all.

Part One | *Early Years*

1 *Beginnings*

ALTHOUGH James Waring left Savannah, Georgia, as a teenager to go away to school and never returned for any lengthy stays, an editorial appeared in the *Savannah Evening Press* over sixty years later, at the time of his death: "For more than 150 years the name 'Waring' has been a bright star in Savannah's medical firmament–shining unfailingly in good health or in the dark days of epidemics now years in the past when it appeared that yellow fever would burn out the city's populace."[1]

The editorial, which appeared on June 4, 1962, went on to eulogize the late James Johnston Waring, M.D., of Denver. Stricken with tuberculosis as a young man, Waring spent much of his career fighting the spread of the disease and supporting the search for new treatments. He also was a devoted educator, leaving his mark on two generations of students at the University of Colorado School of Medicine, and had a reputation as an internist of distinction. He attained national and international recognition for his work in chest diseases. Knowing James Waring's roots helps one understand the man, for family loyalty was important to him, as were his commitment to medicine, public health, and medical history. These allegiances he shared with his grandfather and great-grandfather, both of whom were outstanding physicians.[2]

Great-grandfather William Richard Waring (1787–1842), not wishing to be a planter as were his forefathers, enrolled in the newly established South Carolina College, earning a B.A. degree in 1808. He then went on to the University of Pennsylvania in Philadelphia to study medicine. According to family legend, he had become engaged to his first cousin before finishing medical school but broke off the engagement when, in his medical studies, he learned the relatively new theory that first cousins should not marry. This break-up angered his Charleston kin, and he felt obliged to leave town.

Immediately on graduating from medical school in 1813, William Waring went south to enlist in the army and served along the Georgia frontier in the War of 1812. Three years later, after the war ended, he settled in Savannah and established a practice. He wrote essays for scientific journals and became well known as a man of scientific interests. In 1820 he was asked to make a report on the yellow fever epidemic that devastated Savannah.

William went abroad in 1822 for further training, visiting England, France, and Italy and studying with doctors and scientists wherever possible. In 1826, two years after his return to Savannah, he married Anne Johnston, the daughter of Col. James Johnston, a wealthy banker and merchant of Savannah. The couple had five children.

A yellowed clipping from an unnamed Savannah paper dated 1937 tells of the historical significance of "Dr. William R. Waring, president of the Georgia Medical Society, and in his time the most prominent physician in Savannah"[3] and recounts his interest in the science of meteorology, "making records of temperature, rainfall, direction of wind, etc. and recording the same in his journal, together with observations on the health of Savannah and on the growth of crops on his Skidaway Island plantation." The article observes that Waring's most notable accomplishment was the inauguration of the system of dry culture of rice, which "has had great effect, when properly carried out, on the prevalence of malarial fever in Savannah and vicinity."

This man of many interests went on to serve as both an alderman and as mayor of Savannah, and he was not afraid of stirring up controversy by speaking out. In a speech delivered in 1832 to the Georgia Medical Society, William Waring took the South to task for its poor health habits, specifically among those who overindulged in drinking and eating and those who took little exercise. The speech contained one sentence that came closer to home than Waring could have foreseen: "In marriage [the southern lady] generally breaks rapidly and contracts the appearance of decay or of premature old age from childbearing or from nursing and for the most part dies early." His own wife died four years later at thirty-six, leaving five children. James, the grandfather of Dr. Waring of Denver, was nine at the time of her death.

Education was of paramount importance to William Waring, and his will stipulated that "no expense be spared to give my children the very best education, as I desire them to be well and thoroughly educated." He died in 1842, six years after the death of his wife, and left enough money for the boys to go to school in the North. The eldest, William Jr., had attended Mr. Bolmar's School in West Chester outside of Philadelphia, and James was enrolled at the time of his father's death. James's account (circa 1842) of Fourth of July fireworks at Mr. Bolmar's School is a treasured letter:

I dressed myself as quick as possible, brushed my hair and then put

> my jacket into my pantaloons pocket, you may wonder at my getting into it but it was made of linen and I easily did it, and the reason why I had to do it is because Mr. Bolmar will not let us wash our face and hands with our jackets on, as soon as I had done washing, I ran down into the play room, got my fire crackers, ran to the kitchen, got some fire, and fired off the first cracker. . . . At eight o'clock we set off all sorts of fireworks as a "Flying pigeon," "Sky rockets," "Triangles," "Pinwheels," "Roman Candles," "Snakes," and different other things.

Waring also strongly counseled his executor to invest the children's money in the North, preferably in New York or Philadelphia bank stocks. "I give you this advice because I am convinced of the greater safety and security of property in the non-slave-holding portions of the Union. If they should be obliged to sell any of this property, let it be such as [is] located in the South." He left a plantation on Skidaway Island, near Savannah, as well as other real property and many slaves; and, to "the first of my sons who shall study the profession of medicine," he left his library of hundreds of books. These went to William Jr. The library was eventually bequeathed to Savannah and was placed in the courthouse.

The executors were to supply the children with money "requisite and proper to maintain them decently and respectably in the world, and it is my desire and wish that . . . my children may not be injured by the too abundant supply of money before they can know the proper use of it. . . . After they shall be liberally educated I desire that they be applied to some Profession or Pursuit which may render them capable of acquiring the means of subsistence by their own personal exertions and that they may make them independent of any property that they may inherit from me."

James Johnston Waring (1829–1888), William Waring's second son, was greatly influenced by his father's life and philosophy. In choosing to go to Yale, James was following a tradition of others of his family's position. (William Waring's brother, Alston, had graduated from Yale in 1815.) After graduating from Yale in 1850, James Waring took a medical degree at the University of Pennsylvania School of Medicine. Both father and son served at Blockley Hospital in Philadelphia.

When he finished his formal training in medicine, James went to Dublin and then to London for further medical study. Of this period, his grandson's family possesses two slides. One shows an admittance card for Waring, dated 1853, for St. Bartholomew's Hospital, for "Lectures on General and Morbid Anatomy by James Paget," a British surgeon considered one of the founders of the science of pathology. The other surviving memento of this period, dated 1854, is an admittance card to the Royal College of Surgeons.

After his medical studies, James made a grand tour of Europe with his brother Frederick (known as Fred or Fritz in the family), also a Yale graduate, class of 1852. While visiting with an aunt in Georgia upon his return, James met a shy South Carolinian named Mary Alston, whose father, Thomas Pinckney Alston, owned a plantation. James fell in love with Mary, and the two married and went to live in Washington, D.C., using Mary's dowry of ten thousand dollars to build a house. James joined the faculty of the Columbian Medical College (later known as the National Medical College and eventually as the George Washington University School of Medicine) and taught obstetrics and physiology. Two years later, in 1859, he was elected surgeon and curator of the Washington Infirmary.

In these difficult days before the outbreak of the Civil War, Waring's views were primarily Unionist. Shortly before Fort Sumter was fired upon in 1861, Waring delivered the graduation address at Columbian Medical College, urging that those in science not take part in what was a political conflict. However, in time his sympathies shifted toward the South, and when Mary's father became critically ill, she went to join him, taking with her their three children: Annie, Mary [Mamie], and Alston. Her husband followed shortly thereafter, abandoning house and property. But when he attempted to return, the lines had been drawn, and he was turned back. Returning to Savannah, he offered his services to the Confederate cause and was put in charge of the medical department of North Carolina.

When James returned to Savannah after the war ended to start a practice, his homecoming was clouded by the loss of Mamie, his second child, who had died at five years of age during the war. Not long after his return, he was taken to task by the Georgia Medical Society. A black man who was a patient of his and a legally elected clerk of the superior court asked the doctor, along with others, to underwrite his bond. Waring agreed to help. This action caused an uproar, not only in political circles and among friends and acquaintances but also in the medical society, which first voted to censure and then to expel Waring. He responded by taking the society to court, eventually winning his case in the Georgia Supreme Court. The society reinstated him.

But conflict again came his way. As an elected alderman he worked to make the city healthier, advocating, among other things, a new sewage system. Like his father, he also spoke out against the manner in which rice was cultivated near the city, but old methods for the most part still prevailed. Waring observed that the "wet culture," with its flooded land, caused malaria and yellow fever. Although he did not know the cause of yellow fever, he perceived that the damp conditions contributed to the spread of the disease.

Savannah had two especially severe yellow fever epidemics, in 1820 and 1854. Another one, in 1876–77, took the life of James's brother Fred. James wrote the official report on the epidemic and its possible causes, just as his father had written a similar report over half a century earlier. His 1877 treatise, "The Epidemic at Savannah," calling for drainage and better sanitation, stirred up controversy that brought Waring some criticism. This time public opinion turned around, and no wet cultivation of rice was allowed near the city. It was a victory for James Waring in a cause which he considered his life's work. He died in 1888, shortly before Dr. Walter Reed's work in Cuba in the 1890s proved that the disease was caused by a virus transmitted by mosquitoes.

The house that James Waring bought for his growing family was at 3 Perry Street, near the center of Savannah, a colonial city built on a system of squares according to plans drawn in England by James Oglethorpe.[4] The squares were evenly spaced around a grid. Fronting the squares were the Greek Revival, Georgian, Colonial, Regency and other impressive mansions of the shipping tycoons and cotton barons. Number 3 Perry Street did not face a square, nor was it a mansion, but it was a substantial clapboard house with high-ceilinged rooms and tall windows.

Family historian J. Frederick Waring, with a fine eye for detail, provided a description of the home. In the dining room, French doors led onto a porch, from which wooden steps descended into the garden. A wrought-iron fence surrounded the garden, which had a large magnolia tree and flowering shrubs in brilliant profusion: azaleas, mimosa, japonica, and "birdseye" pepper bushes that provided the little stinging green peppers that James Waring liked in a soup called gumbo.

A daughter, Helen, was born to the Warings during the war, and three more children followed after it ended—James (Jimmy), Thomas Pinckney (known as Pinck), and Mary (Minna)—making six surviving children. In addition to his medical practice, Waring also ran a plantation, "Sedgebank," about five miles outside the city. Although not a wealthy man and subject to recurring financial anxieties, he was able to send his children away to school. He shared his father's views on the importance of a thorough education. The first to go away was Alston, the oldest boy, who went to the Hopkins Grammar School in New Haven and then on to Yale.

By 1877 Anne, the eldest child (born in 1857), had finished school in Virginia and was at home again. Among all the "Ann"s and "Anne"s of her forebears were also some "Annie"s, and this is the name she was known by in the family. Slight of stature, she was a beautiful, vivacious, dark-eyed brunette. In the years after the war she had borne responsibility for the care of her siblings, and now, at twenty, she was attending social functions as a much-sought-after young lady.

When she was twenty-three she met a Spaniard named Antonio Gogorza, or de Gogorza. Born in 1851 or 1852 (his place of birth is listed as Cartagena, Spain, but this could have been his port of embarkation for North America), Gogorza had reached Savannah by 1875, for in that year he appears in the city directory as working for an import-export firm. That he was interested in consular affairs is apparant, for a newspaper notice of July 23, 1875, states that the Argentine and Italian consuls had left him in temporary charge of their embassy business. And he was soon serving as Portuguese vice consul, for on February 1, 1879, an exequatur (an official accreditation for a consular officer) was issued at Washington naming Gogorza a vice consul of Portugal at Savannah. Gogorza, a Mason, had made enough social connections to be listed in the newspaper as a member of the Georgia Hussars and the Georgia Historical Society.

Why Gogorza came to this country at all is a matter of conjecture. According to Basque law, property descended to the oldest child, whether male or female, and many younger sons emigrated as a result. Gogorza had reached the age of military service in the early 1870s and may have been avoiding the wars being fought in Spain from 1872 to 1876. There is also evidence that he may have gone to Cuba with the military in the 1870s and stopped at Savannah instead of returning to Spain. According to a genealogist in Madrid consulted by a descendant, Ruth Waring Halpenny, an "Antonio de Gogorza" was on a roster of men bound for Cuba.

What is known is that Waring did not wish to give Gogorza his charming and highly intelligent daughter, who had many more suitable admirers. But Annie insisted, her parents relented, and the young couple were engaged to be married. At their wedding on February 18, 1881, Christ Episcopal Church was "filled with the beauty and fashion of Savannah," wrote a society reporter. In those days it was not unusual for newlyweds to live for a while with in-laws, and so the Gogorzas moved in at 3 Perry Street.

The Waring household was a crowded one in 1881. It included James and Mary Alston Waring; Alston, twenty-one, when he was home from Yale; Helen, nineteen; Jimmy, sixteen; Pinckney, fourteen; Minna, twelve; and Annie and Antonio. According to family lore, Waring railed at his son-in-law for not working hard enough. Gogorza responded that he had expected a dowry; in Spain dowries were the rule, and he had been distressed that none was forthcoming.

On November 27, 1881, a son—Antonio Johnston, known as Tono—was born to Annie and Antonio in their bedroom at 3 Perry Street. By the time the second son, James Johnston, was born nearly two years later on August 11, 1883, relations between father and son-in-law had deteriorated to the point where they seldom spoke. After dinner Gogorza would go straight upstairs or sometimes disappear for the evening. Waring apparently made little attempt to control his temper, and the women of the family must have been in a constant state of apprehension. Gogorza had a brace of pistols and knew how to use them; he had more than once been involved in a duel. Minna, the youngest child, said long afterward that she had once seen a pistol under his pillow.

By 1884 the animosity between the two men and the tension inside the home had reached the boiling point. Waring ordered Gogorza out of the house and out of their lives, and Annie filed for divorce. The last time the family saw Annie's husband was during that summer, while they vacationed in a cottage in Saratoga Springs, New York. Gogorza, who had been living apart from his wife, came there to see her; when he left, Annie was in tears. For a long time thereafter, Annie slept with the little boys beside her, their nightclothes pinned to hers because she feared that Antonio might try to steal the children while she slept. Divorce proceedings were begun, even though divorce, especially in Savannah's prominent families, was almost unheard of.

When Minna went away to St. Margaret's School in Connecticut the following year, Annie, though only twenty-eight, wrote to her: "When I think of your age, so young, so free of care, so happy (and I pray you may always be so!) I feel in comparison that you are in fact my baby sister. I am so old that I often wonder if I ever could have been young. I don't believe I ever was, even as a baby." The final divorce decree was granted in 1889, eight years after their marriage ceremony, on the grounds of desertion. Annie was awarded the right to resume her maiden name and to change the children's surname from Gogorza to Waring.

Other somber events befell the family during the 1880s. Before the boys had reached mid-childhood, the Waring family lost four members. Annie's younger sister and brother, Helen and Jimmy, died in their early twenties, Jimmy of tuberculosis, Helen of an unspecified cause. Annie and her mother nursed both at home during the last lingering months of their illness. Jimmy was in his senior year at Yale when he became ill—too ill to take final examinations or attend graduation—but his classmates successfully petitioned the authorities to grant him his diploma.

In 1888 James J. Waring, Annie's father, died at the age of fifty-nine. He had been pushing himself hard, as always. Not only was he a busy physician and plantation owner, he also had become a land developer. In the mid-1880s he opened an area that became known as "Waring's Ward." J. Frederick Waring writes that he was involved almost continuously in controversy. His fiery nature contrasted with his warm family side; he told wonderful stories, recited poetry, and played the piano. In the year before his death, he became involved in a charitable project, the Endowment Fund of the Georgia Medical Society.

A couple of years after Dr. James Waring's death, a nephew of his—Frederick Jr. (Fritz)—also contracted tuberculosis and, as he had no living family, he was taken in by the compassionate Waring women at 3 Perry Street. Fritz died in 1891. As always, it was Annie who bore the major part of the burden. With Alston, the eldest son, married and living elsewhere in Savannah, the household at 3 Perry Street now was headed by James Waring's widow, Mary Alston, known to her family as Gamma. J. Frederick Waring's memoir states:

> Gamma was quite small. She always dressed in rustling black, and on her soft gray hair she wore a lace cap. . . . [She was] a shy modest person who . . . lived a long life filled with difficulties and yet [was] still serene and quietly staunch. . . . Of her seven children, she saw one die as a child and two, Helen and Jim, just as they reached adulthood. She lived through the privations of the war and the reconstruction and stood by her volatile husband in all his struggles—on one occasion holding his pistols in the garden while he practiced for a duel, and on another sending the sheriff out to the plantation to stop a duel she did not approve of! . . . I wish I could tell you where such strength came from in so quiet and shy a person.

Mary Alston, who lived to be eighty-seven, "was always the calm center of the family, gentle, firm and brave. All looked to her for guidance, common sense, for the sure standard of integrity and honor. . . . This shy, kindly old lady was a woman of strength, of enduring character."

Like her mother, Annie was strong and resourceful in the face of adversity, devoting herself to the upbringing of her two sons. To support them, she first gave private music lessons at home. When they were older, she taught at a small private elementary school for boys. Among her pupils was Conrad Aiken, the future poet, who, it was said, described years later how much he had gained from having her as a teacher. She also taught Sunday School at Christ Church; Antonio and James became familiar with the Bible. J. Frederick Waring writes:

> I was always a little afraid of Aunt Anne, I suppose because she seemed critical and children are naturally afraid of criticism just as they are afraid of a frown. Once Charles [one of J. Frederick's cousins] failed to put his nickel in the collection plate at Sunday School and afterwards spent it on all-day suckers that left their mark on his mouth. Aunt Anne traced the crime to its root, and Charles has never forgotten the heat of hell-fire and the smell of brimstone.
>
> She expected the best of you and never hesitated to say when you did not show your best. . . . Aunt Anne was as direct as Gamma was shy. She . . . chose instantly between right and wrong, with no hedging and unhesitatingly insisted on the right. Fortunately . . . [she] had a great love for people and great gentleness and understanding. Righteousness without these is often very blind.
>
> When talking with you she gave you all her attention, her head lowered a little and a little cocked to one side, her dark eyes fixed on yours. There was no escape and no desire to escape, unless you had a bad conscience. But it was always best to "tell all" and have done with it and start over again with some of the soundest advice you would ever get.

Antonio and James were brought up by three women, the third being their Aunt Minna, who never married and according to the family was "most scornful of men and very funny on the subject of marriage." Her nephew, J. Frederick, writes that she was devoted to her brothers Pinckney, James, and Alston: "There is no one I know who can think of more nice things to do for people than she."

Despite any sorrow that may have hung over the household, Annie's two boys were well-behaved, easy to teach, and full of interest in life. They were extremely close, sharing the same heavy burden. Sibling rivalry seemed to be nonexistent; they had learned to pull together, given their special circumstances. Loyalty was of paramount importance, and the family closed ranks around Annie and her sons. Both boys were good-looking, with their mother's dark hair and eyes. Unspoken was any comparison of the brothers' looks with the appearance of their absent father.

The education at Mr. Morton's school for boys was mediocre, but Antonio and James had the benefit of their mother's teaching ability and a house full of books. The library at 3 Perry Street was the most used room in the house, with ceiling-high bookshelves on three walls. Mary Alston subscribed to the *London Graphic* and the *London Illustrated News,* which contained fascinating photographs from all over the world. Years later James Waring said of those bound volumes, "I loved them as a boy and I still do." The front parlor, across the hall from the library, was used for more formal occasions and had the best furniture, including Minna's grand piano and a crystal chandelier. J. Frederick tells of the adults talking in the library on Sunday, after church and before two o'clock dinner. In winter a fire would be blazing in the fireplace in the dining room, and in front of it a big plate-warmer filled with dishes awaited the dinner bell. J. Frederick also tells of Antonio's Victrola, and recalls sitting in awed silence as it "scratched out gloriously the first 'red-seal' records of opera we had ever heard." Other mementos, such as the boats James and Antonio had made, were kept in the attic. Their books—"mostly G. A. Henty"—were in their mother's room. A pile of bones that "Grandfather had used in his study of anatomy" was another source of youthful interest.

Sometimes, as they grew older, the boys had a chance to fish and even to hunt. In a letter Antonio sent to his mother when he was at Yale, he drew a little sketch showing "Jim shooting at Faraway," holding a gun, aimed at birds. Relatives probably introduced the boys to these sports. Cousins on the Johnston side were in particularly good supply: William Waring's wife, Anne Johnston, had eleven brothers and sisters. And her father, Col. James Johnston (1769–1822), also had been part of a large family—the first-generation family of Andrew Johnston, who had come to Georgia from England about 1750 as a "practitioner of physick."

At least part of each hot Savannah summer was spent at Saluda, in the South Carolina mountains, where the boys met a new assortment of cousins from Charleston. Gamma had been a Charleston girl, and the children's great-grandfather, William Waring, had originally come from there. William belonged to the fifth generation of Warings in South Carolina. The first Waring in South Carolina, Benjamin, had arrived with a wife, children, and a number of indentured servants from Barbados in 1683. Because he had paid their passage, he was given a certain amount of land to clear, and in time it became a rice plantation. However, the land, located about twenty miles from Charleston, was unhealthy, and in about 1800 Benjamin Waring's descendants moved to Summerville or to Charleston.

Annie Waring, with her interest in history and pride in her family, joined the Colonial Dames Society, but there is no record that Minna ever did, and she was indeed a free spirit. J. Frederick describes her gaiety and her quixotic ways.[5] The garden at 3 Perry Street was her special domain. But Minna would not allow two things: One was being required to go to parties, and the other was having her independence in any way curtailed.

Annie Waring was fully up to the task of guiding her young sons, combining the roles of both parents. A letter she wrote years later to one of her sons gives some insight into the guidance given Annie by her father: "I learned from your grandfather an important lesson. Is your object in life a good one, have you selected the time and place of action? Then brush aside smaller issues and press forward . . . surer that God will help you bend all these energies of yours to the great overcoming of self. So only can you walk with uplifted head, a keen eye, free."

A letter she wrote several years later to James told about an incident that happened when he was still in school in Savannah: "I can see you now, sitting on my bed fighting hard to be relieved from Mr. Lawrence, whom you despised, using every boyish argument known to an ingeniously youthful brain. How I hated to combat your cause . . . [but] the point I was fighting for was too important to let slip. You had to learn tolerance for your own sake and for the sake of your future usefulness." This was a theme she would return to again with her younger son.

Antonio and James were good students, and by the time they approached the last two years of high school they were well qualified for scholarships at a good preparatory school. Following the family tradition of sending children north to complete their education, Annie chose the Lawrenceville School in Lawrenceville, New Jersey. She had taught them well, not just academically but also in lessons of character. Seeing them leave for the North must have been painful for her, but she knew they must have the education that would help them make their way in the world. Antonio left in 1897 and James followed the next year.

Annie Waring's situation was a difficult one: divorced at a time when divorce was scandalous, and a single parent supporting her sons primarily on her teaching salary. Emotional support came, of course, from her close-knit family; her drive and motivation came from special qualities within her and a deep religious faith. But she drew her resilience from another source as well. Born in 1857, before the Civil War began, she had grown up knowing the turmoil many families had endured during the war and recovery. Writes J. Frederick Waring: "The generation of our father and mother had to struggle out of the Reconstruction into a new life that they made for themselves, but they had grown up in the fragments of the old, and the undertones of bitterness and hardship were not missed by the sharp ears of their children, nor the note of pride in the gallantry and spaciousness of 'Before the War.'"

2 | *Achiever*

WITH Antonio enrolled at Lawrenceville in the class of 1900 and James in the class of 1901—"Naughty-One," they called themselves—a correspondence of prodigious proportions ensued. The boys wrote their mother regularly, and she wrote almost daily, letters laden with advice about their studies, discourses on ethics, and expressions of her love for them. Writing in the passion of the moment, she never penned dull letters. She wrote directly, with warmth and vitality and sometimes with stern rectitude when she felt it necessary. Both sons respected and appreciated her advice. They loved her dearly.

Writing in an artistic, stylized handwriting, not always legible, she used dashes excessively, in the manner of that time, a habit James continued. One of the earliest surviving letters in the boys' correspondence with their mother is from Antonio, dated September 18, 1897: "I did a thing the other night that was rather impolite although I didn't mean to." He explains that he was sitting in the parlor with his back to the door listening to three student musicians when some ladies came in. He offered his chair but did not actually get up because a teacher had asked the boys not to move. "That night I was feeling miserable over this. . . . I thought of home and how you would have sympathized with me and given me friendly advice." Antonio was testing the waters of preparatory school, where changing circumstances would try the good manners he and his brother had been taught.

They also had been taught to care about others. A letter to Antonio shows Annie's concern for those who needed help: "At the theater the other night I noticed a small wizened boy handing water up and down the aisles. The play was a modern sensational one and besides the hours being unwholesome for a small boy, he could and did absorb some of the evil in the very air. . . . I get so sick over the children, the poor boys. We scorn them because they are unfaithful in later life and do not protect their impressionable youth." Another: "The little boy . . . whom I taught sent today to say he wanted to see me. He was finally carried to the hospital and Uncle Pinck took off his leg. . . . There is small chance of recovery. Poor little chap."

A number of Annie's letters to James have survived, written in the last months of his senior year, when he was seventeen. One scolds him because she feels he has been inconsiderate. "We all should take care to be courteous in speech and act, and my son certainly." In another she tries to cheer him up after a debate that did not go well for him: "I am glad the debate is over and honest work always counts even if not rewarded with brilliant success. Seize all opportunity for extempore speaking and this want of success may be the means of rousing your ambition in this very line."

"Don't forget Good Friday," she implores in one letter, and in another: "Do be careful about your nose, Dearest, I should hate to have you disfigured. The exercise is all right but do be careful." She concludes, "I'll give you a new baseball shirt if you can wait till after Easter." Sometimes his mother writes to James as if he were a much older person: "Your letter is very sweet and I need your protecting love especially when I feel a little tired." But at other times she treats him like a child: "I must acknowledge I do not like the idea of your getting disobedience marks. You are too old for those and the very name sort of hurts me."

Antonio was named Head Boy of the class of 1900. As when they were younger, there was no sign of any sibling rivalry between James and Antonio; on the contrary, each was proud of the other. Over half a century later the younger brother wrote to Antonio's widow, "I think it is quite too bad that no emblem went with his position as Head Boy at the Lawrenceville School." In the letter in which Annie admonishes James for his disobedience marks, she comments favorably on two articles by Antonio in the Yale literary magazine. Yet apart from this sort of sharing of family accomplishments, no indication is found that she used each boy's successes to spur on the other in competitive fashion.

Like his brother before him, James distinguished himself among his classmates. A letter dated April 10, 1901, enclosed a clipping from the Savannah paper about local boys at Lawrenceville: "Mr. Waring, who is the son of Mrs. Anna [*sic*] Waring, has been chosen valedictorian of the graduating class. . . . Mr. Waring has developed into quite a fine orator and last year won a medal for oratory." Annie offers a suggestion about his coming talk: "A thought has just come to me, do not make your valedictory 'hot air' as you choose to define it but select a theme and deliver a real message, just tacking your farewell on as a 'complement.' What do you think of quoting Hamilton Mabies' theme,'The Ultimate Aim,' then building your own superstructure . . . on the idea of the artist's work and the artisan's!" Along with the letter, she sent him an essay by Mabies, a Victorian writer fond of platitudes, and James referred to it in his valedictory speech.

A month later she writes: "Do not spoil a good record by getting 'even' inopportunely. I warn you. My Boy, be careful. You may go too far. I know you are perfectly true and honorable but 'disobedience' I object to! . . . Think for the moment how mortified you and I should be if you were removed from the Upper even temporarily and it might cost me more than mortification, though I prefer to lose dollars than reputation. I know you well and this is a fair warning to my upright laddie." A week later she was upset because James, after visiting Antonio at Yale, had made his own arrangements regarding a roommate there for his freshman year. "Who is he? Where is his place of residence? I like to know with whom you are to live in such close quarters next winter for many reasons. I have methods of finding out things that you have not."

Finances were an ever-present problem. On April 26, 1901, she writes: "Your Uncle Pinck and I went carefully over your prospective expenses for next winter [at Yale] and he says $4.50 per week for your room is too high, but the reason I think I would prefer your going into a single room is that you can be quiet when you wish. . . . I want you to have good food and comfortable quarters because your health is a first consideration."

Toward the end of May, about two weeks before graduation, James hurt his wrist and could not write. "I am afraid this is a serious accident to your wrist," she writes. "An obstacle is sometimes your best friend. Rise to the occasion and don't hear of 'doleful dumps'. . . . Have your valedictory typewritten if you wish to learn it and do dear child begin to learn it because it's better to speak. . . . Forget the prize, just let them see the grit of the South and I'll be satisfied."

In early June Dr. McPherson, the headmaster of Lawrenceville, wrote a reassuring letter to James's mother:

> I met James a few minutes ago and found him looking tired, but he told me that his hand is improving rapidly. He has developed some little streaks of mischief this year, which to me are of no account. He is one of the nicest fellows in the school and one of our very best scholars. My own son, who is very fond of him, is extremely sorry that they cannot be in the same college.
>
> You need not fear but that he will now come out all right, although his injury and extra work which he has been doing may prevent him from getting what his brother received at the end of his course.

Of the "little streaks of mischief" to which McPherson refers, the only documented incident occurred during the fall of 1900: On election day, James and his entire class went on strike for a half-holiday. The headmaster had decreed classes as usual on that day, but James's class voted unanimously to "strike" and spend the morning loafing about in the countryside. Driven by hunger to return for lunch, the boys then passed a somewhat uncomfortable afternoon, wondering what retribution awaited. Finally, at evening prayers, McPherson passed his sentence: The students were grounded until every boy had made up twice the time he had lost during his morning off. No one was suspended, and Annie's letters do not mention the incident. By today's standards, it seems a tame prank for a class nicknamed "Class of Naughty-One."

As valedictorian, James—a thin seventeen-year-old with big dark eyes, wearing an honorary mantle—gave a serious talk: "We must not hesitate or be afraid when our cue is given to come forward upon the stage. We cannot expect to go through life as easily and as happily as we have through Lawrenceville." Turning to the trustees, he expressed appreciation for their help: "Not for one instance do we repent of having come here. . . . Every contemplated and actual change has been for our welfare." To the masters: "Our lives have become purer and more like those of true Christian gentlemen under your influence." To McPherson: "We appreciate that your aim has been so to ripen our minds and hearts that we would understand that the ambitions of the mere 'artisan' were not for men of our possibilities, but that the ambitions of the 'artist' should inspire us and lead us on to greater and higher things . . . . At all times, we have found in you one to whom we were not afraid to go when in trouble and to whom we were glad to go when in sorrow." Then he turned to his classmates:

> The best life consists not in striving after material gains but in working for the best that is in us, working to give that best to all who have a right to demand it of us, not merely because it is right to do so but because our Alma Mater, our fellow man, our Creator, all expect it of us. . . . I charge you choose your friends with the greatest of care. . . . Though it should seem to be unnecessary, I charge you, be gentlemen. . . . Lawrenceville delights in boasting that we are true Laurentians and a true Laurentian, of course, ought to be a true gentleman.

James then removed his honorary mantle and draped it upon the president of the class of 1902.

Some of James's Lawrenceville mementos have survived, showing his diverse interests. Among the souvenirs are invitations to join the Lawrenceville Calliopean Society, which he accepted, and the Philmathean Literary Society, both known for their debating competitions; a program for a field meeting of the Lawrenceville Association, with penciled notations recording all the winners and their times; a program for Buffalo Bill's Wild West at Madison Square Garden; a program for a Lawrenceville dance; a calling card for a Miss Saidee Hull King; a letter from L. W. Hornblower, managing editor of the literary magazine, offering him the position of associate editor for the 1900–1901 school year, which he accepted; and a program for Washington's Birthday Commemorative Exercises, with the principal address, "What It Means to be an American," delivered by Woodrow Wilson, then professor of jurisprudence at Princeton University.

Also preserved is the menu for the farewell dinner to the class of 1901, a gargantuan feast that included such treats as clams on the half shell, mock turtle soup aux quenelles, lobster à la Newburg, fillet of beef aux champignons, and broiled spring chicken, concluding with strawberries and ice cream, assorted cakes, cheese, almonds, "café, demitasse," and bonbons.

The profile under James Johnston Waring's name in the Class of Naughty-One's year book read: "Call him, if you will, bookmaker, not author."—Voltaire. Editor of Lit.; First Prize Oration, '00; member Calliopean Society; Vice President Y.M.C.A., '01; Valedictory, Class Day." Known to his classmates as "Jimmie," he had jumped from associate editor to become editor of the Lawrenceville literary magazine, which may have been the "extra work" McPherson referred to in his letter to James's mother (and which prevented him from being named Head Boy). In any event, James did not waste time comparing his achievements with Antonio's. He was looking ahead to the next stage in his studies.

FAMILY TRADITION in large part guided James's choice of colleges. His grandfather and three uncles had graduated from Yale, and Antonio had followed in their footsteps. Yale College was celebrating its bicentenary in 1901, the year that James entered college. James, however, chose the newer Yale Sheffield Scientific School rather than Yale College, or Yale-Ac, as it was known on campus. James had long thought seriously about becoming a doctor, and he probably picked the scientific school because "Sheff" offered more courses related to medicine than did Yale College.

The scientific school had been established to promote "the study of the natural, physical and mathematical sciences in Yale University."[6] In John Fulton's biography of neurosurgeon Harvey Cushing, the author writes: "Yale College during Cushing's undergraduate years was in a state of transition from a small and rather self-satisfied teaching institution, which offered social advantages to the sons of its more wealthy alumni, to an institution of learning with graduate schools and a broader university outlook. Yale had also developed in its Sheffield Scientific School a group of men with an outstanding reputation in the field of science."

In *William H. Welch and the Rise of Modern Medicine,* Donald Fleming quotes Welch in saying that as early as 1870 the Sheffield Scientific School offered "a good practical knowledge of chemistry, physics and general biology . . . especially for the preliminary training of prospective medical students." Welch named several distinguished graduates as testimony that "its contributions to a science of great medical and biological importance are unequalled in number and value in this country and have given it rank with the best laboratories of its kind in the world." However, he neglected to mention that it appeared to some as though Sheffield and Yale-Ac were "separate countries on the same planet," as one writer described the two campuses in 1902, although they were only a few streets apart. When James Waring was there, Sheffield had begun to change, but it still had no campus and few dormitories. Like most of his classmates, he lived in a boardinghouse and ate in an "eating-house" where students paid by the week for three meals a day, served at one big table. Sheffield men who were good athletes were accepted on the Yale football and baseball teams, but little mingling took place between the men of the two campuses during leisure hours.

James apparently was not bothered by any lack of social intercourse between the schools. Just eighteen when he entered Yale-Sheff, he was first and foremost a serious student. He was spurred on constantly by his mother, who had little patience with anything that looked as though it would waste time. If he wanted introductions to Yale-Ac students, he had his brother, who was not only an outstanding student but also a social success. In his junior year Antonio was tapped for Skull and Bones, Yale's oldest secret society, established in 1832. When Antonio was later asked to join Phi Beta Kappa, his mother wrote: "Your success is very dear to me," but then later queried, "Now what are you going to do with your 'success'? I have always felt that word does not mean just a prize to hold and grasp and walk off with, but a foundation to build something else on." Because Sheffield men generally were not admitted to this senior society, it seems unlikely that not being chosen would have disappointed James.

Concentrating on his studies in his freshman year, James was like the majority at Sheffield, young men who were very serious about their work with little time for anything else. Sheffield students were not governed by strict rules and regulations such as compulsory prayers and church services, as were students at Yale College, probably because Sheffield students were generally older.

Annie's letters to Antonio are full of suggestions that he look after James. She states that Antonio—considerably shorter than James, who at some point began calling his brother "little Tono"—should take him to call on "Mrs. Townsend and Mrs. Mansfield," two New Haven society matrons with whom Antonio had an entree. She wanted her sons to "cultivate a little outside acquaintance. . . . A man who looks too steadily at himself and his individual aims, his one pet ambition, is apt to narrow his horizons and confine his outlook so that if he receives a shock, his whole vision is distorted and he sees everything black because he won't look beyond himself."

"Has he [James] sufficient exercise and occupation and interest?" she asks Antonio. She wants Antonio to help James with his clothes and to fill in his time "profitably yet with interest." In another letter she expresses the hope that James and Antonio might have Thanksgiving dinner together and that they will be prompt in getting their tickets for sailing home at Christmastime. The steamship line gave a 10-percent discount for Yale, Lawrenceville, and other students traveling together.

At Sheffield the freshman courses were mechanical drawing, chemistry, German, French, plane analytics, calculus, and English. At the end of freshman year, a student had to decide whether he wanted to be an engineer, a chemist, or some other scientific specialist, or whether he wanted to pursue a liberal education. Serious student though he was, James did not always keep his nose to the grindstone. Among his memorabilia he kept a note from the Sheffield Scientific School: "I have been directed by the faculty to inform you that you have been reported absent from fifteen exercises since the beginning of the present term. Three excused, two made up." A copy was sent to his mother; her warning followed.

No evidence exists of any activity involving young women during his freshman year, but his memorabilia for the next two years (Sheffield was a three-year school) included invitations to coming-out parties, dance cards, and pressed boutonnieres. In 1903 he rented a Mexican coat, pants, and sash. A receipt issued four days later bears the notation, "Mexican sash ruined."

A big Yale-blue scrapbook, bulging with mementos, shows that James enjoyed himself in a number of ways. His yearbook entry: vice president, University Football Association; secretary, University Athletic Advisory Committee; secretary, Sheffield YMCA; class deacon; vice-president, Lawrenceville Club; class book historian; Class Book Committee; Class Fund Committee. He was also a member of St. Elmo and of the Southern Club. The caption next to his photograph:

> Is sweet and voluble in his discourse. The blood of this errant rebel boiled first in Savannah, Ga., 1883, and has not yet cooled off. It is perhaps on account of this peculiarity that the corner he occupies in the hearts of his classmates is so well heated. Although a conscientious deacon, the position has not interfered in the least with 'Jim's' popularity. Under the moral obligation of this office, but with a sublime disregard for the truth, he puts down Horse's Neck as his favorite drink. 'Jim' is noted for his black Southern eyes and peculiar exclamatory sounds.

These lines were written by James's best friend at Sheffield, Edward Hall Putnam, nicknamed Ted or "T. Put," from Metuchen, New Jersey. Putnam's yearbook entry described him as "popular with everybody" and "known for his wit and jokes." A note survives in the scrapbook: "The Committee of Leaders has chosen you to lead the Sheffield Religious Meeting Signed Edw. T. Putnam October 1, 1903 P.S. If you are not on hand there will be hell to pay."

A number of theater tickets, balcony section, in the big blue scrapbook attest to James's and Putnam's excursions to New York City to such famous hits of the day as *Floradora, Captain Jinks of the Horse Marine* with Ethel Barrymore, and *Fiddle-dee-dee* with Weber and Fields, Dewolf Hopper, and Lillian Russell. Among the faded and unidentified snapshots one face recurs—that of a puckish-looking young man who may have been Putnam. The scrapbook also contains a card with James's name printed on it with his Yale address (111 Grove Street, New Haven) along with Putnam's, announcing: "We are getting out a 'corking' class-book, containing histories of each member of the class."

James's loyalty to Yale was established and stayed with him throughout his life. By the time he was ready to graduate, in June 1904, he was well educated and socially self-assured, and he knew what his career would be. He continued to profit from the still-abundant advice of his mother. One of the last letters she wrote to him at New Haven was an intense response to some incident in James's life in which he had apparently displayed intolerance toward someone's shortcomings. It was dated June 8, 1904: "I know of no more dangerous indulgence to oneself than to steer off from a necessary contact because 'It's disagreeable.' You notice I said necessary contact and this occurs in one's daily routine—a fellow in class, in society, . . . in the laboratory, on the streetcars, in your pew in church. . . . I know whereof I speak, for I've experienced it. But don't yield to it my son." An even more intense letter followed a week later in which she warned of "the serious consequence of an indulgence in that tyrannical spirit of intolerance." His mother's letter concludes:

> I am going to touch upon a matter of inheritance. Your mother is impatient and impulsive and quick to speak and act but I may add in this cool analysis not intolerant. In truth my grave fault lies in the other extreme. Your father was clever but passionate and intolerant to a marked degree so that you stand between natural inclinations in a position worth studying. . . . Cultivate with all your power of mind and spirit under God's grace the ability to see and hear and feel and speak dispassionately.

Her rare reference to Antonio Gogorza was written from Blue Ridge, Pennsylvania, a place where she went in the summer: "Simply perfect, cool, sunny, green, lovely" is the way she described it. Now forty-seven, she was able to write of the man who had hurt her so deeply, hoping that sharing the knowledge of his father's trait would curb James's inclination toward intolerance. "What are your plans?" she asks, in conclusion. "Is it Johns Hopkins or not decided, for you are free to choose."

"I CANNOT REMEMBER THE TIME I did not want to be a doctor," James writes. "It is a source of great family pride that my great-grandfather, grandfather and one uncle were doctors and that numerous other close and more distant relatives are or have been doctors." And so family pride and tradition affected his career choice, just as it had influenced his choice of Yale. Brother Antonio, undecided up to the end of his Yale years, had enrolled at the College of Physicians and Surgeons of Columbia University in New York City. James's grandfather and great-grandfather had gone to the University of Pennsylvania. James chose to go to the Johns Hopkins University School of Medicine.

The university was founded in the 1870s in Baltimore by Johns Hopkins, a merchant and a Quaker. The medical school opened in 1893; it had been slated to open four years earlier, in 1889, when the Johns Hopkins Hospital opened, but a postponement was forced when the endowment fund suffered reverses. Mary Garrett and other daughters of the Johns Hopkins trustees stepped forward and raised the needed half million dollars, making their contribution contingent on these stipulations: A bachelor's degree or its equivalent was to be required for admission, as was a knowledge of French and German; there would be four rather than three years of instruction; and women were to be admitted on the same basis as men. The high standards embraced by Johns Hopkins ultimately helped to bring about changes in medical schools throughout the country.

Dr. William Osler, who had been on the faculty at McGill University in Montreal and then at the University of Pennsylvania, arrived at Johns Hopkins Hospital in 1889. He helped revolutionize medical education in the United States by creating its first medical clinic along the lines of clinics in German medical schools. Another innovation was the introduction of clinical clerkships, which brought the student into the wards. Further, Osler introduced resident staff, another idea borrowed from German clinics. At this time, U.S. hospitals had only interns, who usually served just a year. Unlike U.S. or English hospitals, Johns Hopkins had both a chief of medicine and a chief of surgery, who devoted the greatest measure of their time to the hospital. Osler made bedside teaching important, with practical instruction to small groups of students. Until this time, large amphitheater lectures had been the rule.

James entered Johns Hopkins in 1904. What influenced his choice is not known, but the attraction of attending an innovative institution must have been a consideration. In eleven years the medical school had become renowned for the caliber of its faculty, its advanced form of teaching and the active role it offered students in their training. There may have been other factors, such as the links between Yale-Sheffield and Johns Hopkins: Daniel Coit Gilman, the first president of Johns Hopkins University, had been involved in the founding and development of the Sheffield Scientific School. The reputation of the Johns Hopkins faculty also would have been appealing. Osler, a Canadian, was in the last of his sixteen years on the faculty when James arrived in the academic year of 1904–1905 to begin his studies.

"The Chief," as Osler's colleagues called him, had accepted a call to occupy the prestigious Regius Professorship of Medicine at Oxford University, where he would become Sir William Osler. He was renowned for his comprehensive medical textbook, *The Principles and Practice of Medicine.* Teaching was Osler's foremost interest, and he addressed the young people before him as "fellow students." James's correspondence with his mother does not tell whether he ever sat in a class taught by Osler; however, the great man's aura permeated the medical school. Osler, described as being tolerant, religious, self-controlled, and a good listener, had a great capacity for work and showed great concern for patients and students.

One of Osler's colleagues, professor of pathology Dr. William Welch, was instrumental in bringing Hopkins to the forefront of medical education at that time. He brought a group of bright investigators with him when he came to Hopkins. Noted portrait painter John Singer Sargent was commissioned by Miss Garrett in 1905 to paint a portrait of the "Famous Four": William Osler, medicine; William H. Welch, pathology; Howard A. Kelly, obstetrics and gynecology; and William S. Halsted, surgery. The picture, which shows the celebrated quartet assembled in their academic gowns, was presented by Miss Garrett to the university on January 19, 1907, during Waring's junior year. The four were remarkably young for their eminence: When called to join the hospital in 1889, Osler was thirty-nine; Welch, thirty-eight; Halsted, thirty-seven; and Kelly only thirty-one. A few months later he became head of obstetrics and gynecology.

Of the four, only Welch is mentioned in James's surviving correspondence with his mother. James discusses him in a November 1906 letter to his mother, written late in the evening after the fraternity to which he belonged, Nu Sigma Nu, had taken the professor into its membership. Director of the most famous teaching laboratory for pathology in the United States, he was affectionately called "Popsy" by his students. James told his mother of how the professor had held the fraternity enthralled for several hours after the regular meeting with his stories of the history of medicine: "I think if somebody asked me what opportunity in an educational line I would like to have, I should unhesitatingly reply: 'Let me eat where he eats, above all let him take an active interest in me'. . . Such profound knowledge on every subject under the sun. Undoubtedly he is the greatest man I have ever known. God bless 'Popsy' Welch." Ultimately, however, it was Osler who most profoundly influenced James, as attested by ex-students, colleagues, and family.[7]

But James had other mentors. Below the level of the "giants" was a faculty member who picked him out from the bevy of bright students and took a special interest in him. Dr. Lewis Hamman of the Department of Medicine, in a letter to Dr. Gerald Webb of Colorado Springs, written after James had left Hopkins, pronounced James to be "the most promising student" he had seen there. The young man never forgot his encouragement; fifty years later he contributed to a memorial scholarship fund at the Johns Hopkins medical school in honor of his teacher. "I can never forget Louis Hamman's interest in me as a medical student," he wrote. "I treasure his memory."

James found the intellectual atmosphere of Johns Hopkins stimulating, thanks in great measure to the excellent faculty and students of high caliber. Between his love for his medical studies and his drive to excel, he was unable to slow down. He pursued virtually no interests but medicine after entering Hopkins in 1904. Occasionally he indulged in sports, as revealed in a Christmas card he received years after his graduation from medical school in which a former classmate recalled a memorable game James had pitched for the medical school baseball team, probably in the spring of 1906.

In the summer of 1906, after completing his sophomore year, James worked at a hospital for crippled and deformed children at its summer quarters in Blue Ridge Summit, Pennsylvania—in what capacity is not known. Letters have emerged over the years from Annie to her sons with this return address, for she went there regularly for the summer. James and Antonio played baseball on a team made up of college players who were summering in the area. James was the pitcher, according to yellowed clippings in the big blue scrapbook.

Blue Ridge Summit also represented a bittersweet significance in James's life, for here he kept company with a young woman named Edith Duer. Letters Annie wrote to Antonio a few years after 1906 make it clear that James had met a girl for whom he cared deeply. Her family was from Baltimore and summered at Blue Ridge. Waring's busy and overworked schedule left him no time to follow his heart. Years later, in 1958, he received a letter from Edith's brother, Leland, a lawyer in New York City, telling of her death. The letter closed: "I should love to see you and talk over old times at Blue Ridge."

In September 1906 James plunged into third-year studies back in Baltimore. His letters to his mother were conscientious, often quoting Marcus Aurelius, whose deep devotion to his own mother and brother James understood. "In my Marcus Aurelius," he wrote, "I have underlined these words: 'From my mother I learned piety and beneficence and abstinence, not only from evil deeds, but even from evil thoughts;

and further, simplicity in my way of living, far removed from the habits of the rich.' And, 'I thank the gods for giving me such a brother, who was able by his moral character to move me to vigilance over myself, and who at the same time pleased me by his respect and affection.'"

A letter from Antonio in November 1906 shows the strong bond between the brothers. Antonio, in New York City at the College of Physicians and Surgeons of Columbia University, told how busy he was, of his need for perspective and of his need for his mother and James. "It is good to feel, though, that the connection between the three is an elastic one. Distance stretches it and tightens it so that we feel its force, distance never breaks it. . . . I just want you always to feel that I am here 'with the goods' and that my love for you is an unfaltering one and will never fail."

Stirrings in the devoted younger son showed that he needed to have some freedom to think things through himself, as in this letter to his mother: "I feel sure there never was a mother who gained so completely the loving confidence of her young sons as yourself . . . and yet the workings of a boy's brain are more strange and curious than those of any other piece of machinery in the world. And every boy has to 'mark out his own technique' in some things. I was no exception to such a rule."

Although ostensibly referring to his youth, it appears that his emotional development lagged behind his intellectual maturity at age twenty-three. His total immersion in his work is evident. As the third year progressed he wrote:

> My dispensary work comes so much nearer being the real thing that it interests me continually . . . Already my "intolerance" is beginning to show itself. In the dispensary yesterday I was told to remove a tumor from the back of a little girl's head. A classmate was instructed to give the ether and a nurse to hand the instruments. Mark this—the other fellow had never given ether in his life. The nurse was worthless and I knew powerful little. The man who should have stood by and supervised the process disappeared. Well—the girl is alive and the tumor was removed but Providence and the little sense I had are the only reason why. That dispensary doctor, in my opinion, is not worth the salt in his bread and it would give me a great deal of pleasure to tell him so. Fortunately I am spared contact with him most of the time and I am slowly learning not to allow my real feelings to be spread out like an open book on my face.

In light of Annie's earlier missive to him on "the tyrannical spirit of intolerance," it must have helped him to confess to her.

So intent was James on his studies that it was no doubt frustrating not to be able to take advantage of everything else that Hopkins had to offer. It was more than just the excellence of professors that made the atmosphere exhilarating. Drs. Welch, Osler, and Billings formed the Historical Club to pursue the history and bibliography of medicine. Osler also founded the Journal Club to keep up with current medical literature and formed the Laennec Society for studying tuberculosis in all its phases. As a junior medical student, however, James's time for outside interests was severely limited. As the year went on, a note of frantic compulsion became evident in his letters.

> March 8, 1907:
> I want to do so much better than I do . . . disappointments in myself discourage me sometimes in a manner that demands all my little philosophy and common sense and grit to spur me on to yet greater efforts rather than waste time in morbid introspection and self-blame. My ignorance on many points I count no great shame, because we cannot know everything, but the failure to reason correctly and quickly, to appear more ignorant than what I am because of what I may call psychical inhibition is very trying. . . . You should never lose the clue to my thoughts, Dubbie [his childhood name for her] for that would mean that you do not understand me and that would break my heart for I count on you always for that.

Two days later he told her that, as much as he would love to come home for Easter and "just loaf around," the nine examinations coming in May were "of supreme importance." Just how hard he had been driving himself became evident:

> Since Christmas I have devoted myself to my work with all the powers I could command, have pushed myself to do things that it seemed hardly possible my weary brain could get down to. I have gone to church Sundays, and then, sad to relate, worked over half the rest of the day. This against your counsel and against my desire most certainly, but to me it seemed necessary. Those few hours bind the connecting links together of facts that I must know. . . . Slowly, oh so slowly my mind builds up the mental picture of disease after disease that every hour, no, every minute I must needs devote to anything great or small that will help to complete

> my knowledge of medicine. Possibly I have been absorbed too much in my work, I know it would be healthier for me to do this or that instead of working, but I came to the conclusion long ago that a medical student with any ambition loses a great deal of his common sense while he is in medical school.

What James did not tell his mother was that he had not been feeling well; that he had been having night sweats, coughing, and low fevers; and that he had consulted a doctor. Ten days later, Annie received an envelope from James containing two letters. The postmark was March 20, 1907; the return address, Johns Hopkins Hospital. The first letter:

> My dear brave Mother,
> In the enclosed letter I am going to make a demand upon your bravery. I warn you here—for it was an awful hard letter to write and I want you to be brave as I am. I love you so very very dearly that I want to spare you every possible care and worry and it grieves me deeply to have to add another care to your too many already.

Then came the second letter:

> My dear dear Mother,
> Once more I must turn to my Marcus Aurelius for philosophy. That great emperor said, "Misfortune well-bourne is good fortune"—it shall be so for me. Do you remember a letter I wrote you a few days ago and a promise I made in that letter that when anything serious turned up I would let you know myself at once? Well Well—I felt very sure at the time—no occasion would arise to write you serious news. It seems I was wrong. It is a hard job dear Mother, but listen. You know I do not talk of you to many fellows but I have to Bill. I told him my trouble today and spoke of you and he said, "She has Faith—which means so much." It's the early bird that catches the worm my dear Mother, and I am one of the earliest of the early birds and consequently have everything in my favor. In 15 years science has advanced much and particularly the Science of Medicine. To this great advancement in science and its improved methods of diagnosis and treatment I am indebted to knowing just where I stand today. And given that chance that 15 years ago Uncle Jimmie and Fritz Waring did not have. Is not that a great deal to be thankful for—I feel sure you will say yes. But my—what a shame that those two fine young fellows should have been taken in

the flower of their youth—simply for lack of what the Medical Profession knows today—while I—less worthy than they—God knows, can profit immeasurably by it and can still look on life with a smile on my face and my teeth gritted and say "not my will but thine". . . .

I just learned about it today though I had suspected for ten days, but was confident that Dr. Cole would let me know as soon as they found out. . . .

A few râles in my left lung and a few tubercle bacilli in my sputum—a little fever and you have the picture of your earliest case. That's the word we must bank on Mamma the word we must encourage ourselves on—earliest—earliest—every chance yet Mother dear—every chance—and I am glad for I would hate to have to give up now.

It means I have to lay off at least a year—but what's a year? Talk with Uncle Pinck about it and come to me when you can—and I hate to be selfish but I must have you with me for many a solid month off some place in the mountains. . . . These men have been honest with me—I have demanded it—and in less than ten days I'll be on my feet to wander with you anywhere you say—to fight it out for health and strength—you and I with little Tono adding his prayers and our trust in God and it all will come right. God bless you and keep you dearest and best of Mothers,

Your devoted son,
James Johnston Waring

Even before finishing the first page of this letter Annie would have guessed that James was talking about tuberculosis, but in those days people were reluctant to name that terrible and often fatal disease. It was then the greatest cause of death. Only toward the end of the letter did James refer to "tubercle bacilli" and "rales," an abnormal rattling sound in the chest, audible through a stethoscope, typical of tuberculosis. When James's physician, Dr. Rufus Cole, wrote to Annie, he did not mention the frightening word, either.

It is very hard to write to you about your boy, for I know the news that he has written you is going to be a great shock and is going to cause you a great deal of distress.

But it isn't as bad as it probably seems at first and while it means his giving up the rest of this year, I hope he is going to get well again very quickly. The trouble is in a very early stage, and

> with the right kind of care and direction I trust he will improve very fast. . . . I feel very hopeful and I do hope you will be able to take this view of it.

Consumption was the name then most commonly given to tuberculosis, or phthisis, as its pulmonary version often was called, and the prognosis was grave in early decades before chemotherapy was developed to control it. James was putting on a brave face, but, reading between the lines, it is clear he was devastated.

3 | *Slough of Despond*

TUBERCULOSIS is a bacterial disease caused by the organism mycobacterium tuberculosis. Most tuberculosis is acquired by the inhalation of bacteria-laden droplets from the cough or sneeze of someone with the active disease. It can affect almost any tissue of the body, although in the vast majority of cases it attacks the lungs. The name "The White Plague" was given the disease in reference to the white cheeselike substance in the pulmonary cavities. It may have another connotation as well—one pulmonary physician attributed the name to the paleness of victims.

The disease is one of the oldest known. Prehistoric bones have been found that show its effects; Pott's disease, tuberculosis of the spine, has been found in skeletons six thousand years old in Egypt and Peru. The Israelites knew of it: "The Lord shall smite thee with a consumption, and with a fever, and with an inflammation" (Deut. 28:22). In the second century B.C., Galen, a Greek physician who was renowned in Rome, sent his consumptive patients to an area on the Bay of Naples for the climate, prescribing milk and inactivity.

Rest and good nutrition remained for centuries the best regimen physicians had to offer consumptives. But little more was known about tuberculosis until the mid-seventeenth century, when Michael Ettmuller first attributed the spread of the disease to sputum (expectorated matter made up of saliva and secretions from the respiratory passages). In 1683 Leeuwenhoek, inventor of the microscope, described bacteria, a milestone for medical science. An Englishman named Benjamin Marten wrote in 1722 that "minute living creatures" were the cause of tuberculosis, but he was ignored. Leopold von Auenbrugger in 1761 developed a new method for detecting heart and lung diseases by tapping upon the chest. "Percussion" was popularized by Corvisart in the beginning of the nineteenth century. This technique enables the physician to determine the density of underlying tissue, an air-filled lung making a hollow sound, and a solid, or fluid-filled, diseased lung emitting a duller note.

Then came René Théophile Hyacinthe Laënnec, who in 1818 invented the stethoscope, with which the physician listens to the passage of air through the airways. Together with percussion, this process, called auscultation, enabled doctors to determine much of the pathology in a lung. In this era before x-rays, lungs could be seen only at autopsy. Laennec postulated correctly that phthisis in its many forms—of the spine, lungs, and others tissues—was one disease. He wrote *Diseases of the Chest* (1826), laying the foundation for modern knowledge of tuberculosis and other chest diseases.

In 1862 Louis Pasteur formulated the germ theory of disease, founding bacteriology, opening huge vistas of understanding of the causes of disease, and leading to preventive inoculation. In Paris in 1865, Villemin proved that tuberculosis could be transmitted from man to animal and from animal to animal. He called the infecting organism a "germ," now known as a mycobacterium. In the same year Joseph Lister in Glasgow, Scotland, treated his first patient with his antiseptic surgical techniques.

The modern treatment of tuberculosis began in 1882, when the German doctor Robert Koch isolated the tubercle bacilli and proved beyond doubt that the disease was contagious. Koch, using the theories of Pasteur, tried but failed to effect a cure with a potion made of dead tubercle bacilli. Although Koch "lymph" could not protect against the disease, it was useful in diagnosis: Small quantities injected into the skin would produce a transient swelling in an infected patient but no reaction in a healthy person.

In 1895 Wilhelm Roentgen's discovery of the x-ray revolutionized medicine and proved invaluable in diagnosing tuberculosis. And in the very year that James Waring became ill, 1907, another German, von Pirquet, introduced a simple diagnostic skin test based on the concept of allergy in tuberculosis. Thus, in the two decades since Waring's young uncle and cousin had died of this disease, advances had been made that might, through early diagnosis, have prolonged their lives and that everyone hoped would save James's.

At the time James Waring acquired the disease, the annual death toll from tuberculosis in the United States was about 200,000. It was the most common cause of death in this country and in Europe. Indeed, a diagnosis of tuberculosis was equivalent to a sentence of death. Decades later, a former classmate who knew of Waring's condition and had heard nothing of him since medical school days suddenly discovered that he was still alive. He wrote, as Waring described it, "a nice congratulatory letter which began, 'Good God, Jim, I thought we had buried you thirty years ago!!'"

The disease's symptoms included weight loss, fatigue, fever, and night sweats. In pulmonary tuberculosis the tubercle bacilli, inhaled in droplet nuclei of sputum or in dust, are drawn into the air sacs of the lungs. The body reacts by building around the focus of bacteria a wall of scar-like tissue, or granuloma. The bacteria, however, do not lie dormant within this casing but necrose its core. When it becomes sufficiently soft or liquid, this tissue is coughed up or spread to other parts of the lung via the airways, eventually forming cavities within the substance of the lung. As the disease progresses, the victim coughs blood, which may lead to a massive hemorrhage and death. Although the process is self-limiting in most people, in some the disease, apparently inactive for many years, may reactivate spontaneously without a new infection; in others the disease may spread beyond the lungs to other parts of the body. The disease also occurs from drinking milk containing bovine tubercle bacilli, causing an infection frequently outside the lungs, usually in the bones or lymph glands of the neck (scrofula).

The myth arose that the disease was prone to attack people in the arts, for among its most famous victims have been writers, poets and musicians: the Brontës, John Keats, Voltaire, Ruskin, Percy Bysshe Shelley (who actually died by drowning), Ralph Waldo Emerson, D. H. Lawrence, and Frederic Chopin, to name a few. Was it true that the disease affected a disproportionate number of the creative members of society? No. The explanation seems to be that lettered people were more affluent and could afford to see a doctor and pay for a diagnosis; they also wrote and described illnesses.

Another myth arose that the disease was inherited, a view held by Hippocrates. Tuberculosis became a stigma, thought to be connected with some hereditary defect, and attitudes about the disease were fatalistic. Claimed Dr. René Dubos in *The White Plague* (1952): "The factors which determine susceptibilities or resistance to tuberculosis are controlled by heredity, become modified by living conditions and have as their basis some of the processes of immunity." Dubos did not imply that tuberculosis is a hereditary disease—which it is not—but maintained that heredity may influence the complex immune responses of an individual, determining his or her susceptibility to the disease.

The disease flourished in crowded cities. As standards of public health rose and nutrition improved, the disease began to wane. Among the factors considered important in 1907 as influencing the development of tuberculosis were diet, climate, and mental state. Osler said that the fate of the tubercular depended more on what "was in his head than what was in his chest." There was one theory that the obsessive-compulsive personality was at greater risk than other personality types. James Waring, in letters to his mother, described himself as having become obsessive-compulsive about his medical studies.

Although it will never be known precisely just how he contracted the disease, one explanation is that he may have been infected after performing an autopsy. Doctors who knew Waring had heard this theory; one recalls that Waring told him that four students had worked on a cadaver at Hopkins and three subsequently died. Tuberculosis could be transmitted in the anatomy laboratory because embalming does not kill bacilli. Furthermore, in working on the wards at Johns Hopkins Hospital, where many poor patients were treated, Waring must have been exposed frequently to pulmonary tuberculosis, both diagnosed and undiagnosed.

Thirty years after Waring contracted the disease, a study made in 1937 by Dr. J. A. Myers and others on approximately 12,000 university students showed that "the number of students enrolled in the schools of nursing and medicine is a relatively small group, yet there is an overwhelming preponderance of lesions in this minor group, indicating to us that the problem of tuberculosis among young adults is most acute among those students who, while in the line of duty, come in contact with tuberculous patients. . . . There were 85 cases of pulmonary tuberculosis found among the students studied, and of these 73 [86.9 percent] were either in the school of nursing or were premedical students who had contact with tuberculosis patients."

Another explanation as to how Waring became infected comes from Anne Waring Maer, his daughter. She heard that a cook in the boardinghouse where her father lived may have passed on the disease. Or he might have been exposed in the summer of 1906 while working at the children's hospital in Blue Ridge Summit. Another possibility is that he had been infected at home, as a child, and that the infection had lain dormant ever since.

When Annie Waring arrived in Baltimore in the last week of March 1907, her main concern was not how her son had become sick but how he was to become well. The doctors at Johns Hopkins recommended the sanatorium* established by Dr. Edward L. Trudeau at Saranac Lake,

---

*The word was spelled both ***sanitarium*** and ***sanatorium*** at that time. The first comes from the Latin *sanitas*, meaning health; the second from the Latin *sanare*, to heal. Trudeau chose the former, but ***sanatorium*** generally became standard for a hospital for treatment of chronic diseases, as tuberculosis, while ***sanitarium*** was used for an institution for the promotion of health, a health resort. ***Sanatorium***—the spelling preferred by James Waring—will be used hereinafter unless the word is incorporated in the name of a specific institution.

New York, in the Adirondack Mountains.[8] Trudeau's Adirondack Cottage Sanitarium was the first of its kind in the United States. Robert Louis Stevenson had gone there twenty years before Waring—also with his mother—seeking a cure for his lung disease. At the time of the Stevensons' arrival in 1887, Trudeau's sanatorium was expanding from the original single cottage and two-patient capacity to a larger facility.

Trudeau had nursed his brother Francis in the late 1860s, often sharing his bed in a tightly closed room, at a time when tuberculosis was not known to be contagious. After Francis's death Trudeau enrolled in the College of Physicians and Surgeons of Columbia University in New York City. His health deteriorated steadily; but only in 1872, after he was married and trying to establish a practice in the city, did he finally see a doctor. The outlook was grim: He had tuberculosis, and the upper two-thirds of his left lung was affected. At that time, the only recognized treatment for the disease was a change of climate. There was no consensus as to what climate was the best—the only recommendations were to live in the outdoors and, many believed, to exercise frequently. Only the well-to-do could afford to be sent away.

After showing no improvement during a winter in South Carolina, the young doctor stayed in Saranac Lake, and, to his surprise, his health improved. But after he returned home to his wife and two children on Long Island, his health failed again, and the four of them returned to Saranac Lake to a rented house. Despite the cruel winters, when the temperature could fall as low as minus 40 degrees Fahrenheit, he decided to live there permanently. After a few years, he was well enough to take patients, and having read about the success of sanatoria in the mountains of Germany and Switzerland, he decided to start one himself.[10] The first cottage, "Little Red," was ready for patients in 1884 and was incorporated in 1889.

By the time of Jim Waring's arrival in 1907, Trudeau's Adirondack Cottage Sanitarium was considered the best of the approximately 100 in the United States. More patients applied than could be accommodated, and only those with a substantial hope of improvement were accepted. Recovery was not a word much used by Trudeau; if he could "arrest" the disease, he felt that he had done his best. Trudeau believed in prescribing rest and was one of the first in this country to advocate this treatment instead of exercise. From then until the advent of antituberculosis antibiotics, rest remained the cornerstone of treatment.

James and his mother left springtime behind in Baltimore and, after a long and tiring train journey north, found winter still lingering in Saranac Lake. The sharp easterly winds, mud, old snowdrifts, cold rain, and sudden snowfalls were a chilly welcome to the cottages, grouped around a central hospital and administration buildings. Waring was put to bed at once, and his mother found a room in the village, where boarders were welcome in many of the Victorian-style houses.

Waring's year at Saranac Lake was severely trying. "During the first year of my illness," he later said of his time there, "I was the damndest psychoneurotic that ever took refuge in the Adirondack Mountains." A paper he wrote years later ("Differential Diagnosis in Pulmonary Tuberculosis," 1942) described his disability: "The sense of fatigue associated with pulmonary tuberculosis is a deadly thing. It needs to be experienced to be appreciated. It clings relentlessly by day weighting the feet with lead and the back with heavy burdens. It goes to bed with its victim at night and gets up with him in the morning."

Like Waring, Dr. Lawrason Brown, the medical director at Saranac Lake, had contracted tuberculosis in his third year at Johns Hopkins. Brown had gone to Trudeau's sanatorium in 1899. Although he may have empathized with his patients because of this experience, the routine was unbending. Trudeau believed in the beneficial effects of fresh air and sunlight. For eight months Waring was under strict orders to rest and sleep wrapped in blankets on an open porch by day and in a room with wide-open windows at night. Nothing short of a major winter storm with howling winds gave any respite from the regimen, which Trudeau had copied closely from the sanatoria of Europe. Trudeau took credit for being one of the first to advocate the rest cure, and he said he "had to stand my share of abuse about it." Dr. Herrmann Brehmer of Germany believed in gentle exercise; his patients were urged to walk uphill and rest upon benches on their way home.

Three large main meals were served each day at Adirondack Cottage, as well as three other regular "light repasts" and milk, hot if desired, upon wakening at 7:30. There were set times to be out of doors in a chair or bed, morning, afternoon, and evening, if the weather was good; there were set times for exercise, too, if prescribed. Bedtime came after snacks at 9:00 P.M. Large meals were common in those days among the middle and upper classes, and the European sanatoria had been retreats for that strata of society. The underlying rationale was that abundant food was necessary to help the patient gain strength to combat the disease.

Though he chafed under the restrictive routine at Saranac Lake, Waring had significant experiences there and made lifelong friendships. Lawrason Brown became a friend. Allen K. Krause, a member of the class of 1907 of Johns Hopkins, was diagnosed as having tuberculosis in 1908 and went to Adirondack Cottage. His stay may have overlapped Waring's; they later became good friends. Krause became a well-known teacher and editor in the field of tuberculosis.

In "The Fifty-five Trudeau Medalists (1926–1980)," L. Fred Ayvazian wrote, "Often the staff doctors and nurses were themselves at only a more advanced state or recovery—sometimes an important bond." He told of those who became leaders in the field of tuberculosis, fashioning "a seeming tragedy in their lives into stepping stones to service and accomplishment."

"In my very first interview with Dr. E. L. Trudeau," Waring later recalled, "he said to me: 'It takes a bit of the Divine Fire to get well of TB.'" Waring told his students, "I was just another lunger, in a village where there were hundreds, just a miserable medical student eating his heart out with bitter disappointment, frustration and self-pity, and this great physician knew it and came to my help."

"Things were not going too well with me and I was woefully depressed," he later recalled, for he had failed to make progress despite the tediously scheduled care. Just before Christmas, a letter arrived from Trudeau that pleased and touched him so much that he kept the letter all his life and often read it aloud to students.

Saranac Lake
December 23rd 1907

My dear Warring [*sic*],

At this Christmas season I wish I might be able to say a helpful word of cheer to you. To see one's health shattered, one's good ambitions ruined, to be held day by day through long months in the grip of a relentless foe and to be helpless and at times hopeless is hard indeed, but I have known all this and for this reason I can feel for you.

Neither you or I can solve the great mystery of life and its contradictions, perplexities and suffering. I have lived much longer however than you have and have learned that many of the things we so repine at losing are really of little moment, are unenduring and unsatisfying and that to know God in our hearts is what really matters most in this life. I have seen souls grow while bodies shrivel and the really great things of life unfold to a man when all that the world prizes most has been denied him. At any rate I want you to know that you are in my thoughts on this Christmas day and that I pray it may bring you a glimpse of the heavenly vision and that faith and peace and hope may come to your soul! Most sincerely yours

E. L. Trudeau

Trudeau later said that when he wrote this letter, he thought Waring was going to die. But his words, from his experience and given out of kindly concern, had the effect of bolstering the young man's courage. Lawrason Brown, Trudeau's longtime colleague, wrote of Trudeau's "personal charm, his optimism, his wonderful, never-flagging enthusiasm and his love of people. . . . His life was centered in his home, his sanatorium and his laboratory."

Why did Trudeau single out James Waring among hundreds of patients? Undoubtedly he befriended many, but their correspondence shows that Trudeau had taken a special interest in Waring. Beyond sharing the same disease, beyond the appeal of the bright, sensitive medical student, there may have been another, more melancholy, side to their friendship. "I do not believe that Dr. E. L. Trudeau ever saw his father after he was three years old," wrote Brown in "Trudeau's Family Tree—A Study of the Genealogy of Dr. Edward L. Trudeau." Trudeau's father, Dr. James de Berty Trudeau, from a prominent New Orleans family, left his wife and his two small sons, Francis and Edward—like Waring, he was the younger of the two—after eight years of marriage. He returned to New Orleans, joined by the boys' older sister. The boys and their mother stayed on in Paris, where their maternal grandfather was a physician. Having grown up in homes without fathers may have contributed to the bond between the two men.

Trudeau was subject to deep depression because of the severity of his recurring tuberculosis. In a paper written many years after his stay at the sanatorium, Waring wrote, "We know that he suffered almost daily for thirty-odd years from symptoms of the disease." Yet it is Trudeau the optimist who is remembered. In "The Value of Optimism in Medicine," Trudeau's presidential address at the Eighth Congress of American Physicians and Surgeons, May 2, 1910, he said: "The one thing that seems to stand out as having been most helpful to me, and which has enabled me more than anything else to accomplish whatever I have been able to do, seems to have been that I was ever possessed of a large fund of optimism." He pointed out that it was optimism that enabled him to build his sanatorium.

"Very early in my association with [Waring] in the National Tuberculosis Association," recalled Dr. Theodore Badger of Harvard University Medical School at a seminar in Colorado honoring the life of James

Waring, "we were discussing one evening the matter of a cure for tuberculosis. He said that his [time] at Trudeau [was] the best education he really ever had in medicine. He learned and acquired then a philosophy of life which lasted him throughout his entire career. I think it was this perhaps that gave him such an extraordinary insight into human nature."

During his last few months in Saranac Lake, Waring was allowed to live with his mother in a rented house. He was not making the progress they had hoped for, however, and of this period, he later recalled, "When . . . I found myself at the end of seven months still with a most unstable temperature, I was most profoundly discouraged." His mother must have been very worried, judging from the following response to a letter she had written to Dr. McPherson at the Lawrenceville School:

> May 8, 1908
>
> My dear Mrs. Waring,
> Our hearts are all sore about Jim. At nearly every meal, when we are alone as a family, we talk about him and you, your mother and your sister. For all of us have a singular love for him. . . .
>
> I think of my hope and pride in Jim's career, and of course it hurts to imagine, even, that it is not to be realized; yet I do hope that he shall live to a good old age. Yet I am comforted by the thought of what Jimmy is, of which nothing can bereave him, you, or me.
>
> Faithfully and respectfully yours,
> A. J. McPherson

Waring later referred to the "Slough of Despond" into which he dropped while there. Many years later, in "Relapse in Pulmonary Tuberculosis (1923)," he quoted Lawrason Brown: "Roughly speaking, the average graduate of the average sanatorium has about one chance in two of living five years, one in four of living ten years, and one in seven of living fifteen years. If the disease is as active on discharge, he has about three chances in one hundred of escaping death from tuberculosis."

Given those odds, it would have been easy for Waring to have lost all hope. One day Dr. Edward Baldwin, described as "a rather dour, pessimistic individual" by a former colleague, went to see Waring, who asked him if it would do him any good to go to Colorado. Baldwin replied, "You can go out there if you want to, but you're not going to get well, anyway." This response was typical of Baldwin—who, as a student, had diagnosed himself as having tuberculosis—but it awakened something in Waring.

The patient was ready for a change, and his mother, in particular, felt that the long winters of Saranac were too relentless. They said their good-byes to the staff. "I . . . owe a great debt to them [the medical staff at Saranac Lake] for the example they set me of thoughtful, patient attention to my real and also my fancied woes," he later wrote. But Baldwin's prediction that he was "not going to get well anyway" made Waring more determined than ever to win his battle against the disease. In hopes that he would make progress in a higher, drier climate, he and his mother, joined by his aunt Minna and brother Antonio, would journey West by train. Their destination: Colorado.

Part Two | *Starting Out*

4 | *New Beginnings*

TOWERING above Colorado Springs is Pikes Peak, part of the Front Range of the Rocky Mountains—a glorious setting. It is doubtful that James Waring was able to appreciate the panoramic view, for he had to be taken off the train on a stretcher. He and his mother had left Saranac in May 1908 and made the arduous three-day journey with the help of his aunt and brother.

None of the first places Annie and Minna looked at met the needs of the patient, so they went to the Antlers, the best hotel in the city. There they were told that the management could not accept a guest on a stretcher. Faced with a barrage of Southern charm, however, the hotel relaxed the rules and permitted James to be whisked upstairs via the freight elevator. Not long after, he entered Cragmor Sanatorium; Annie and sister Minna found a house to rent. "The change of scene," Waring wrote later, "and a new doctor—Dr. Swan—brought me out of the Slough of Despond in which I had dropped and from the third week of my arrival in Colorado . . . I have had hardly a sick day from my old trouble." He must have written an optimistic letter to Trudeau, because in September of that year the doctor wrote to say, "It was good to hear from you again and to hear that you were better. I hope you may now emerge from the dark waters, plant your feet firmly on the bank and gradually come to life again as I have done so many times."

Cragmor Sanatorium, opened in 1905, was not the first sanatorium in Colorado Springs—the Albert Glockner Memorial Sanatorium opened in 1890—but it was the first to be planned on a grand scale. Dr. S. Edwin Solly, a champion of the benefits of climate in the treatment of tuberculosis, was the driving force behind the founding of Cragmor, but his grandiose plans had to be greatly scaled back by the time the sanatorium opened. Solly died in 1906, and the institution was going through a difficult time during Waring's tenure as a patient (1908-1910). In its beginning years Cragmor had a good reputation; it also was expensive, reflecting the luxurious facilities, the food, and the service. Annie Waring was determined that her son should have the best in care and comforts to help regain his health.

Waring's care was under the management of a committee of doctors, one of whom was Dr. Gerald B. Webb, an Englishman in general practice who was becoming a specialist in tuberculosis and was one of the physicians in charge of Cragmor. He had come to Colorado Springs because his American wife had tuberculosis (she subsequently died). Webb and Waring soon became friends, sharing an intellectual curiosity about all manner of things, especially medical history. Webb had an interest in the research of lung diseases, tuberculosis in particular. Waring had arrived well recommended, for Lewis Hamman told Webb that he had been the most promising student he had seen at Hopkins.

In the opening years of the twentieth century, Colorado Springs was attracting people from all over the country and even from abroad. Word had spread about the town's dramatic setting below the grandeur of Pikes Peak, its well-planned layout, wide streets, and shade trees.[10] After gold, the economy of the city was bolstered by the arrival of health seekers and tourists. In time, the city became a mecca for consumptives, sent by their doctors back east. An early account of consumption in Colorado comes from Isabella Bird, an intrepid Englishwoman who toured the Front Range by horseback in the autumn and winter of 1873 on her way back to England from the Sandwich (now Hawaiian) Islands. In *A Lady's Life in the Rocky Mountains,* she tells of visiting a ranch at Plum Creek between Colorado Springs and Denver: "There was a lady there from Laramie who kindly offered to receive me into her room, a very tall, elegant person, remarkable as being the first woman who had settled in the Rocky Mountains. She had been trying the 'camp cure' for three months and was then on her way home. She had a wagon with beds, tent, tent floor, cookingstove, and every camp luxury. . . . She was consumptive and frail in strength."

The notion of using tents as a place of recuperation for consumptives received its greatest push from Dr. C. F. Gardiner of Denver, who conceived of the idea after spending a winter night with a Ute family in their tepee. Gardiner patented a tent that had a wooden floor, a wood-burning stove, and an umbrella-like cover over the smoke hole to keep out rain and snow. Several of these little villages of tents surrounded some of the sanatoriums in the Denver area.

At the end of the nineteenth century, books were extolling Colorado's climate as an ideal one in which consumptives might regain their health. Stated a 1903 Chamber of Commerce publication: "Colorado Springs, a city of 25,000 inhabitants, with an altitude of 6,022 feet, offers . . . the greatest all-around advantages of any place in this country. Its days of perpetual sunshine, its charming life . . . its environs, hospitable people—everything done for the invalid by those who are now cured makes it stand foremost to my mind as an ideal place."

Dr. Charles S. Denison had come West to Denver from New England because of consumption and had recovered. In "The Climatic Treatment of Consumption" (1883) he stated: "To my mind, . . . climate is the most potent means known at the present time with which to combat this destroyer, consumption." The dryness of the air, the number of hours of sunshine, and the temperature variability were all cited as beneficial.

Although many eastern physicians sent their tuberculosis patients to seek relief in Colorado's altitude and sunny climate, other doctors were urging that consumptives stay home. Said Dr. Sherman Bonney: "There can be no greater error than the sending of hopeless, indigent patients to health resorts." Many Coloradans were urging that consumptives stay home, too. The Newport of the Rockies was not looking for more lung patients, and as more and more arrived, some hotels, boardinghouses, and restaurants put up signs reading: "Consumptives Not Accepted." The afflicted tried to get around this prohibition by pretending that they had some other disease. As one of them wrote, "It was surprising the number of diseases I found represented [in his boardinghouse]. But it was more surprising that everyone coughed—dyspeptics, rheumatics, nervous wrecks, kidney patients, ear patients, Keely cure patients [alcoholics] all coughed. For fear of being detected as a consumptive, no one exercised any of the simplest sanitary precautions, so I voluntarily left that hotbed of disease, giving the landlady ten days' notice and getting in return quarter portions of food at the table and no change of linen in our rooms."

This is not to say that there were not charitable people in Colorado Springs, sympathetic and helpful physicians, and boardinghouse keepers who ran sanitary and friendly establishments. In the early days of the influx, local opposition to the health seekers had not yet begun to form; this only came later as worries arose about the contagiousness of the disease. The unsanitary practice of some of the victims in disposing of their sputum by spitting in the streets was also responsible for much of the hostility toward consumptives. Yet nobody doubted that Colorado Springs and its citizens profited from the city's popularity among tuberculosis patients. The avarice of some Coloradans was denounced in Thomas C. Galbreath's *Chasing the Cure in Colorado* (1907): "Colorado is most glad to welcome the contents of the purse the invalid brings with him, but she would greatly prefer that the invalid should not accompany the purse." A victim himself, Galbreath made the case that the invalid would be better off not leaving home in the first place.

Letters to Antonio from Annie, and occasionally from James, tell of none of these horror stories. Waring did not suffer the prejudices experienced by the poorer health seekers. Moreover, he had family support and a new set of friends.

At Christmastime 1908, Waring sent Trudeau a small painting, which Trudeau described in a letter of thanks as "a picture of poor humanity looking for the light of the star." He called it "very striking and full of meaning specially to those of us who live so very near 'that vast forever' and need the light at every step. I will have it hung in my office and it will be most cheering to look at on many days as 'the shadows lengthen and the evening comes.' I am so glad to hear of your renewed health and strength. This must have been a very different Christmas to you and your good mother from the last one when the light seemed dim indeed."

Sometime in 1910 Waring improved enough to be able to join his mother and Aunt Minna in their little house. In the Sexennial Record of the Yale-Sheffield Class of 1904, he wrote, "Have built a bungalow, keep the finest bunch of laying hens in Colorado, weigh fifteen pounds more than I ever have and fully expect to return to work in September 1911, when I shall enter the third year of the Denver and Gross Medical School in Denver, Colorado." These plans would change; he instead would enter the University of Colorado School of Medicine, also in Denver.

Living at home, Waring rapidly grew stronger and often joined parties of other recovering young people for picnics or rides in the Garden of the Gods, a cluster of spectacular rock formations near the city. Annie, despite her anxiety over her son's health, lived a much more enjoyable and cosmopolitan life than had been possible in the remote and austere village of Saranac Lake. In the spirit of the West, the local residents were willing to accept newcomers; the ponderous formality of the East was largely absent. "There is a straightforwardness and naturalness about these people which do not long tolerate sham or subterfuge," wrote George B. Price in *Gaining Health in the West.* "Although the newcomer is usually assured a hospitable welcome, it is always advisable for him to take with him two or three letters of introduction from people of his own social standing, if this is possible." Annie mentioned in her letters to Antonio that she had been given letters of introduction.

Aside from the English set and Americans from both East and West, there was a distinct Southern set. Mrs. Gerald Webb (the doctor's second wife) was a granddaughter of Jefferson Davis, the late president of the Confederacy, and her parents were social leaders in Colorado Springs. Annie and Minna, with their array of Charleston and Savannah connections, may have had introductions to some members of this social clique. They were also acquainted with the Gilpin family, whose daughter Laura, eight years younger than James Waring, would go on to become one of the great western photographers. Gamma, now approaching eighty, came to stay for a while. "You never saw anything like this beautiful summer," Annie wrote Antonio, "so cool and lovely. No excuse not to feel well."

As James's health improved, Annie worried about his trying to do too much. In the summer of 1910, he was invited on a hunting and fishing trip to Jackson Hole, Wyoming, by his friend Lawrence Lunt. Lunt, who grew up in Colorado Springs, was about to enter Harvard Medical School when he and Waring met, and the two had many interests in common. Annie was relieved when Waring's doctor said he was not strong enough to make the trip. She was just as glad when another letter for her son came from Trudeau, indirectly advising caution. "I was glad to see your handwriting," he said, "and to hear such good news of your health. The fight with tuberculosis is often a long one (as I know from personal experience) but when one is on the up grade things look much better and I hope before long you will be on really solid ground and able to 'do things.'"

A few months later, Waring must have written Trudeau about some problems he was having, perhaps more spiritual than physical. Trudeau answered on December 23, 1910, with an unusually long letter telling how he dealt with his own lifelong invalidism:

> My dear Waring:
> Your letter has just come and is a great pleasure. I am specially glad to have you tell me I have been helpful to you and to have you tell me of your difficulties. . . . How often the great mystery of life and its meaning staggers young men who until they come to a great happening or sorrow had never thought at all! . . . Some men and specially some women (I am thinking now of Grenfell [Sir Wilfred Grenfell, who headed a medical mission to Labrador] and my good wife) at once attain a faith so strong & that come what may it is never staggered. Others of us go on struggling & fighting for the light which at one time floods our life and at others is but a spark. Grenfell's faith is an inspiration to me because I knew him personally and his faith is the result of experience: on that floe he

> told me he had no fear and slept most of the night though he expected to die at any minute! One may question his beliefs but no one can question his sincerity!—alas all of us do not attain to such faith but the glimpses we get of the light keep us battering on through life and to many peace & light come at last. . . . I hope it will be so with you. I have long ago ceased to question or try to explain the mystery of existence and its great meaning but I am more & more impressed with the great love in the universe which is struggling for expression. . . . At present I am a little better and more comfortable but I have become a regular invalid (with a nurse) and all the miseries which go with the last stages of TB and an infected bladder. . . . I am better and happier here than anywhere else now that I am so sick the rays of the setting sun glow with the new warmth & the new joy my good friends bring to me all the time.
>
> With every good wish for the New Year,
>
> Affectionately,
> E. L. Trudeau

The envelope enclosing this letter is well worn; it appears to have been carried around a long time in a pocket and extracted frequently. Here was the greatest of the sanatorium doctors carrying on a lengthy correspondence with a young man in the West, not a perfunctory note but a baring of the soul. Despite poor health, Trudeau was able to take some pleasure in life for a few more years. He died in 1915.

The Warings spent nine more months in Colorado Springs, with James steadily becoming able—and eager—to do more and more. His eagerness still troubled his mother, who wrote to Antonio, "Jim has been doing society pretty heavily the last month. Some of it is good and refreshing and wholesome, but some of it here is trivial and degrading and makes one feel a real dissatisfaction and proper discontent. This has been Jim's state of mind recently. Oh, dear lad, he needs, and so be it, if it's God will for him, a man's interests and a taste of a man's occupation if his strength holds out."

Another letter deplored what she regarded as the unseemly frivolity in Colorado Springs among "the Broadmoor crowd" (Broadmoor is an area south of the city, where many socialites lived). There were bets that a lady could not take a man "pickatuck" and dump him into the pool. "Bets kept running high until they bet $100 . . . and she did actually take him across and dump him into the water. Now what do you think of that? Pure idleness here leads people into undignified things."

Annie also disapproved of the lack of compassion afforded the Native American population. Describing a carnival held in the Garden of the Gods, she said that "about twenty-five of the old Ute Indians up here [were] camping on their old grounds. . . . It is quite pitiful to see how we have treated the Indian—made him leave his own beautiful ground here and gave him a reservation in Utah he can't make a living out of. The widow of Ouray, the old chief, was entertained here. . . . [She] was the Chipeta who was kind and friendly to the poor Meeker women after the massacre of the men of their family, yet she is old and no one has been able to move the government to give her a small pension."[11] Jim also became concerned about American Indians, developing a lifelong interest in their history and culture.

Overall, Annie's impressions of her new home were favorable. "I know so little of this place because we have to go slowly behind a horse and can't afford to travel, but it's a wonderful place," she wrote, praising Colorado to Antonio. On the day before James's twenty-eighth birthday, she reminded Antonio: "Tomorrow is Jim's birthday and I do hope you will write him a really godfatherly letter of advice as to his work and living in Denver. . . . We go on September 6th [to Denver, Jim to start classes at the University of Colorado School of Medicine], his porch to fix up and screen but think if I write ahead, can get the workmen on Thursday." South-facing sun porches had become common additions to homes in Colorado with the influx of so many consumptives seeking the advantages of fresh air.

The hoped-for letter from Antonio with "godfatherly" advice has not been preserved; nor would James have resented such a letter. But the letter Annie wrote Antonio five days later shows that her son might have chafed a bit under her surveillance: "Here I am, 10:30 at night, sitting up . . . , as Jim would say 'drooling,' but waiting for him. He has gone to the casino [the Broadmoor Casino on Cheyenne Lake] for dinner." Antonio's letter did his brother "a world of good," and she advised Antonio not to get into debt by buying an auto, as one of his uncles was wont to do.

When his doctors told Waring he would be able to return to medical school, he was overjoyed. "The bungalow has been definitely rented—$75 per month for eight months from October to June," Annie wrote Antonio in July 1911. "Tuesday Aunt Minna is planning to go to Denver to see about houses." Annie wrote that she must live economically in Denver and get the best location, good air, and an extra room for Gamma and Minna. Annie was not in the best of health during this period. She was a small, fragile-looking woman who carried herself well, pinned her gray hair into a bun on top of her head, and only wore gray or black, according to J. Frederick Waring's family history. Swan told her to slow down, to imitate an ordinary hack horse that never allowed itself to be hurried nor worried no matter how prodded. With her usual courage she was soon immersed in plans for the move to Denver, a much bigger place than Colorado Springs and a city where she and her family knew no one.

Antonio was now working with his uncle, Dr. Pinckney Waring, in Savannah, where he would become the city's first specialist in pediatrics. His mother wrote to him before leaving Colorado Springs, "Jim is really anxious to begin some steady work. He said yesterday that the accomplishing of any worthy effort gives one confidence in himself and excites respect from outside besides adding an unconscious poise and dignity. He added sadly, 'You see, I have done nothing and I feel it.' He knows and I know the hard learning of the last few years. But God counts that, not man, and we always, like children, want praise from one another. I value that, too. Indeed I need it as much as anyone, but man isn't free until he can do things without praise."

The Denver that drew James Waring to medical school in 1911 had grown far beyond the frontier town it had been in the previous century. This time Waring was not arriving on a stretcher, as he had in Colorado Springs, and could appreciate the panorama of mountains to the west of the city.[12] Denver was now a metropolis of over 200,000. Since 1904, the city's forward-looking mayor, Robert Speer, a tuberculosis victim from Pennsylvania, had been giving away trees to residents who would plant and care for them. Between 1904 and 1912 he gave away more than 100,000 trees. The most prominent building in Denver was the State Capitol, constructed of Colorado granite and crowned with a brilliant gold-leafed dome.

When the Warings arrived, Denver was undergoing further beautification, with plans developed by master planner Frederick Law Olmstead, Jr., for a civic center, more parks and parkways, and a system of parks in the nearby mountains. Landscape architect S. B. DeBoer, a tuberculosis victim from Holland who came to Denver seeking a healthier climate, began to lay out flower trails in the parks and along the parkways and introduced a wide and unusual variety of trees. "I've been really pleased with Denver, a beautiful open city," Annie wrote Antonio in July. "Will move September 1. School opens September 11."

An exciting spirit of progress filled the air; the Warings had come to Denver at a pivotal time in the city's history, just as it was a historic time for medical education in this country. That James Waring had the right qualities for the coming era in medicine would be proved in the future, but in 1911 he was only an ambitious, hardworking, and rather frail medical student trying to recover from a terrible ordeal. Trudeau wrote: "What a pleasure it was to hear that you are to finish your medical course and get your M.D. after all, for then any number of new possibilities in life are open to you."

Annie Waring "thought and worked and prayed" over her search for a house in Denver and found one that suited her at the same price (seventy-five dollars a month) she had been paying in Colorado Springs. Although it lacked the sleeping porch her son required, she persuaded the landlord to improvise one on an upstairs veranda. Annie wrote of the house: "A small, extremely neat convenient house in excellent locality in sight of Cheesman Park on a lovely terrace, lovely lawn, back and front." The Waring sisters joined a church. To Antonio: "I went to an early service at St. Barnabas just around the corner from us. . . . It is somewhat high-church but such a dear, small chapel and so near."

James enrolled at the University of Colorado School of Medicine, repeating his third year. Established at Boulder in 1883, the school had recently merged with the other medical school in Colorado, the Denver and Gross College of Medicine, and now held all its third- and fourth-year classes in Denver; the first two years were still held in Boulder.[13]

The entire medical world in the United States was feeling the effect of widespread reforms initiated in 1909 by the Carnegie Foundation for the Advancement of Teaching. In that year the foundation had assigned Dr. Abraham Flexner, with one assistant, to visit each of the nation's 155 medical schools and evaluate their standards. The Flexner Report, appearing in 1910, was the result. Flexner's intention, although never fully realized, was to reduce greatly the number of medical schools. Out of the 155 then in operation, he proposed to save only 27!

The Denver and Gross College of Medicine, run under the auspices of the University of Denver, received relatively low marks. The college had been formed in 1902 by the merger of two so-called proprietary medical schools—one affiliated with the University of Denver and the other being the Gross Medical College. (The designation "proprietary" referred to the fact that the school was solely dependent on fees from students for funding. Gross took its name from Samuel D. Gross of the Philadelphia Academy of Surgery.) The report on Denver and Gross commented that not even a high school diploma was required to get in; that none of the instructors gave their full time to teaching; and that the school had no resources other than its fees. Moreover, the document said, "There is a total absence of scientific activity. The rooms are poorly kept. A few cases of books are found in the college office behind the counter," and the dissecting room had only a few cadavers, "as dry as leather." "For hospital facilities," the report continued, Denver and Gross "depends largely on the county hospital, the management of which is political. Clinics are held daily from 8:30 to 10:00, purely through courtesy." Students from all schools merely "look on"; they are "not much at the bedside." Obstetrical work was limited, postmortems rare. Hospital staff appointments were obtained through "pull."

Flexner had kinder words for the University of Colorado's medical school in Boulder, but still wrote that "the University hospital is entirely inadequate." The university's higher overall grade was not surprising, for the American Medical Association awarded the school an A rating in 1910. In that year the entrance requirements increased from a high school diploma to a minimum of sixty hours of college credits (two years). This prerequisite resulted in a decrease of 60 percent in new enrollment.

Flexner recommended the consolidation of the two medical schools, asserting that Colorado contained too many doctors (more than twice the national doctor-to-patient ratio); the state, therefore, "can safely go to a higher standard [of admissions]." By the time his report went to press, however, medical men in Denver already had effected the merger. A constitutional amendment was passed in 1910 permitting the university to teach medicine in Denver. After 1912, the state required that "all applicants for license must have had, previous to their medical education, a year of college work." (The reduction in the requirement from two years of college credit to one year was a response to the shrinking number of matriculants to the medical school.) In raising the standards for training and educating physicians and eliminating those schools that did not meet them, Flexner permanently altered the U.S. medical profession. Because only the brightest and most talented and dedicated students would survive the now-rigorous training, the general public soon came to respect doctors more than ever before.

Waring rode the trolley car to Thirteenth and Welton streets, where classes were held at Archer House, once a private residence. He was taking eight subjects, none of which he had studied at Johns Hopkins, including gynecology, orthopedics, pediatrics, nose and throat, tractions and dislocation, and ophthalmology. Four days a week his classes began at eight in the morning. As he wrote Antonio, this schedule made

> a long day for half a man to start at 6:40 and get home about 4:30 and have about twenty pages of Osler [presumably his *Principles and Practice of Medicine*] to work up for a searching quiz for the next day. I was never strong on working up things in cold blood and writing on them; and I tell you what, Bo, I am some dud at it. The fellows are a rough, profane, blasphemous outfit—noisy—altogether a prep school outfit. . . . Alas for Jonny Hopkins. Them was the happy days. Some days I think this school is not disappointing for I did not expect much. I shall probably learn more surgery than at Hopkins where I learned none and perhaps a systematic study of Osler will do me no harm though I prefer the Johns Hopkins way of studying medicine myself.

In the fall of 1911, to Antonio: "Rather than do too much, I will skip one or two courses and take them with half my fourth year next year and the remainder of my fourth year two years from now."

As the school year progressed, their mother wrote Antonio that she was concerned about James's health. "He has been steady and brave but his mouth takes on a pathetic look sometimes that goes to my heart. He took a bad cold running around in the heat and dust. His first cold for two years. . . . [It is] hard for him to sit in a crowded, poorly ventilated room. He flushes easily. He is surely not strong but has a good spirit, and . . . he had gotten to the point at the Springs of needing some definite interest." A few days later: "He may, after all, have to drop some subjects and trust to making up later if he finds he simply can't move around as the other fellows." He had joined the Denver Athletic Club, where he could have lunch and sometimes rest between classes.

After her first rosy impression, Annie found it hard to get used to Denver, which she thought lacked the gentility of Colorado Springs. Her letters reveal that during her early days in Denver she would have been glad to return to Savannah, where Antonio was living in the old Waring house with his grandmother (Gamma) and had just gone into pediatric practice with his Uncle Pinck. "Nothing could hold me here but Jim's medicine," she wrote. "I get perfectly exhausted trying to find places and see signs and street names and numbers. Certainly it seems strange I should be landed in a big pushing western city when I just love a little place and to be close to a few people, but if this is God's place for Jim, then he will give me the strength and sense enough to do my part." On a cheerier note, she was glad to report, "Our neighbors are gentlefolk and have welcomed us and we know a few others. This is a quiet pretty street, though many of our neighbors are prosperous enough to have machines [automobiles]." One thing Annie had adapted to was the climate of Denver, especially the summers with cool nights and low humidity.

But in general she seemed overwhelmed by her new surroundings. "Denver is such a big, huge place. It gives me a pain though I will say it is not New York. . . . My head buzzes nearly all the time. I can hear it as if I had taken an overdose of quinine." She also complained about the social etiquette—or lack of it—in Denver. In the South, newcomers waited for calls from those who already lived there. But here, no calls were forthcoming. "It's funny, but it's certainly their loss," she stated. "I don't mind being lonely or indeed I shall not be." A doctor in Denver who had been at Hopkins told Waring, "Well, Jim, it's up to you. Come to see me if you want to know us," to which Annie responded, "That's West, I suppose, or selfish or what you will. I hate to say Dr.–like."

But after a couple of months, things began to improve. Annie reported that some friends had moved to Denver and that "we have a few old acquaintances." A while later she wrote, "Jim loves his work and whistles over it and just seems to thank God every day he is able to work. How would that strike a loafer?" In this same long letter she hoped that Antonio would fall in love with "a good, fine woman who can be your real comrade. . . . When I realize what Edith Duer was [the girl Jim had been seeing at Blue Ridge the summer before he became ill] and that Jim cared for her a great deal, I wonder if he will ever find someone quite so nice."

James and Edith must have been good friends, because when he became ill the Duer family went out of its way to be kind to him and to his mother. Edith by now had married, and Annie asked Antonio, "By the way, did you notice that wedding at all? I hope you sent a telegram. . . . It would hurt Jim if you didn't. . . . Don't forget people who stood by your brother as they did. We had a time over Jim's wedding present to her. . . . Life startles me wide awake every now and then and the longer I live, the more I lighten my baggage. In other words, the fewer things I really value or want, but I always want my children." She urged Antonio to write a medical article. Sometimes, her advice was questionable, as when in another letter she urged Antonio to make surgery his specialty: "I believe it will save you too hard a life."

Aunt Minna and, in the beginning, Gamma lived out West with Annie and James, but in the winter they returned to Savannah. Their servant Anna returned to Colorado Springs to stand the Civil Service exam. "I have a Texas girly for whom I am very thankful," Annie told Antonio.

Nobody was more thankful than James Waring, simply to be alive and able to resume his medical education at last. The late Dr. Robert Stearns, who served as president of the University of Colorado (1939–1953, with time out for active duty with the Army Air Force during World War II), reminisced about James at the Waring symposium in 1963.[14] Stearns graduated from the University of Colorado in 1914 and later went on to law school at Columbia University. "I remember him very well as a student. All of the students then were together in Boulder. The place was smaller then, and we all knew each other. All of us knew Jim Waring as a very happy and joyous person who didn't dwell upon his difficulties but, rather, helped us in many ways to overcome ours." If Stearns's recollection was correct, Waring possibly went to the Boulder campus because the Denison Memorial Building was the only place to do research. Henry Denison, Waring's former classmate at Hopkins who had urged him to come West, had died tragically in 1912 while working on a chemistry experiment. His mother, Mrs. Charles Denison, donated his scientific equipment to the Boulder school, along with funds to construct the building, which contained laboratories and other research rooms.

James Waring graduated from the University of Colorado School of Medicine with the class of 1913—one hundred years after his great-grandfather, William R. Waring, had obtained his degree from the University of Pennsylvania. The class contained fifty graduates, including four women.[15] Despite earlier misgivings about the western medical school, he had changed his views. Five years after his graduation, Waring was quoted in the medical school's executive faculty minutes and paid high tribute to the teaching in the University of Colorado as he had experienced it as a student. He did, however, stress the imperative need for more clinical teaching, especially in medicine during the third year.

After graduation, Waring interned for eight months in Denver at St. Luke's Hospital, and then did his residency at the Agnes Phipps Memorial Sanitarium for five months in 1914. Located east of Denver on the present site of Lowry Air Force Base, the facility had opened in 1904 and was well equipped; Lawrence Phipps had spared no expense in founding the institution, which honored his mother. The fees, however, were beyond the reach of most victims of the disease. Dr. G. Walter Holden, the director, was a disciplinarian who expected as much of himself as he did of others under his supervision. He made calls on his patients even during the blizzard of 1913.

The family gained a new member in December 1914 when Antonio married Sue Winburn. The next year Gamma died. She had held the family together, according to J. Frederick Waring's memoirs. After her death the house at 3 Perry Street was divided, with offices in the basement. Alston, a brother of Annie, lived in a little apartment on the garden; he was a widower, and his three sons were away at school.

In 1914 Waring became a part-time instructor in medicine at the University of Colorado School of Medicine. He also served on the staff of the dispensary for tuberculosis outpatients. Both positions were unpaid, and so, seeking to enter private practice, he became the associate of Sherman Grant Bonney, a prominent Denver physician whose specialty was tuberculosis.[16] Bonney, a native of Maine and a graduate of Harvard Medical School, had come to Colorado in 1890 because of his wife's illness. There were no sanatoria in Denver at that time and, seeing a need, Bonney established inexpensive camps for them, including a large one in Estes Park, where groups of patients lived in cottages and received nursing care. He belonged to the "super-alimentation" school of treatment for tuberculosis, which meant stuffing patients with large amounts of food, especially eggs, rare meat, and milk. This mode of treatment was even then in question and later was discredited. Bonney had been professor of medicine and dean of the medical department at the University of Denver and trustee and president of the Gross Medical College of Denver, and when the Colorado medical institutions merged in 1910 he was made professor of medicine emeritus of the University of Colorado School of Medicine. In 1908 he published a pioneering book, *Pulmonary Tuberculosis and Its Complications.* He had a large practice in tuberculosis, as might be expected.

For a young physician who wished to become a tuberculosis specialist, Denver was the place to be. However, the people of Denver expressed some ambivalence, if not outright opposition, to their city's role as "Tuberculosis Capital." The sight of so many sick people being carried from the passenger station on stretchers was unsettling. What happened to them after that often depended upon how much money they had. Good accommodations and treatment were waiting for those who could afford it. For others, the situation could be desperate. As in Colorado Springs, many hotels and boardinghouses feared contagion and displayed signs: "No invalids." Others were more explicit: "No TB patients allowed." Not until 1914 did Denver open its first free dispensary for tuberculous outpatients; Dr. Johanna Gelien volunteered her services and served as its director. One of the first of the residential facilities in the state was the Oakes Home in the Highlands area of northwest Denver, which was opened in 1894 by the Reverend Frederick W. Oakes of the Episcopal Diocese, but he did not call it a hospital or sanatorium. The establishment of the National Jewish Hospital for Consumptives in Denver, which opened in 1899, could be said to mark the beginning of the proliferation of sanatoria in Denver. With "None who can pay can enter—none who enter pay," as its motto, National Jewish solicited support nationally; patients came from across the country. When the hospital could no longer accommodate all those requesting admission, the Jewish Consumptives' Relief Society was formed in 1903, providing facilities mainly for Denver's Jewish community in advanced stages of the disease.

Among other facilities in the Denver area that opened in the first decade of the century were the Evangelical Lutheran Sanitarium in Wheat Ridge; Swedish National Sanatorium south of Denver; and the Bethesda Hospital, provided by the Dutch community. James J. Waring, M.D., placed his name, along with others, on a list of backers of another Denver sanatorium, Sands House. When the first house burned down in 1915, another was acquired to the west in Jefferson County. A letter among Waring's effects told that Sands House was a place for tubercular young women, established by Ida French Sands and organized through St. Barnabas Church, which was his mother's church. The letter also stated that Annie Waring was "one of half a dozen ladies who helped."

Eventually, as many as 200 sanatoria dotted the Denver area, but for various reasons relatively few victims actually went to them, whether because of availability, cost, or dislike of the treatment regimen.

Gradually, laws were passed forbidding spitting in public places and ordering the fumigation of rooms where patients had died. Two proposals that did not pass would have prohibited kissing or handshaking in public. The stigma attached to the disease was such that the words consumption, and then tuberculosis when it supplanted the other, were almost banned from Denver newspapers. This stigma also applied in other cities. In San Francisco, for example, all mention of the existence of consumption had been suppressed to such a degree as to jeopardize the safety of the entire country, according to Dr. Harvey Cushing in his biography of Osler.

As in other places, because of the stigma attached to the disease, people often hid their sickness: the numbers who came to Colorado because of the disease cannot be documented. Estimates are that, at the time Waring came to Colorado, as many as one out of three people in the state were either patients with active tuberculosis or family members of victims. Not only the patients but also the doctors themselves were coming to Colorado because they or a member of their families had the disease. In Denver, where the influx of consumptives from other parts of the country was greatest, it claimed more lives than the next three leading causes of death combined.

Racing to make up for lost time, Waring threw himself into his work, keeping a precarious balance between his work and his health. Dr. E. Stewart Taylor, professor emeritus of obstetrics/gynecology at the University of Colorado School of Medicine, recalled that Waring told him he "rode a bicycle around to see patients at twenty-eight sanatoria when he was a young man in practice." He wrote to his mother, vacationing in Savannah in the winter of 1916, "I sometimes deplore my devotion to my work and my absorption in it, but let it be said that I know and appreciate what to me is the greatest thing in the world and that is the certainty of your devotion to me." He was still living with his mother and aunt in the house they had bought at 1229 Race Street, not far from where they lived when they first arrived in Denver. It was a two-story house on a pleasant block. Judging by the houses near it that still stand today (an apartment house now occupies the site), it was a typical "Foursquare" or "Denver square," a boxy style of architecture common early in the twentieth century.

Waring contributed to the Denver Medical Society library and was its librarian while it was in the Metropolitan Building; in 1916 he was on the library's fundraising committee. The following year he was elected to membership in the Denver Clinical and Pathological Society, an association of leading practitioners in the city. Founded in 1892 by Drs. Robert Levy and C. Fleming, the group held meetings from 1910 to 1920 in the old Grill Room of the Brown Palace Hotel. For the next five years the society met at the Cactus Club in the old Wolcott mansion, located on Glenarm Street four blocks from the Denver Athletic Club. (The group returned to the Brown Palace until 1950, when it began meeting at the Denver Country Club.)

Who nominated him for membership in the Denver Clinical and Pathological Society? One likely person is Henry Sewall, who asked Waring if he might propose him for membership in other societies. Sewall (1855–1936) had earned a Ph.D. in physiology from Johns Hopkins in 1879, which then had no medical department. In 1882 he went to the University of Michigan, where he headed the department of physiology. His ground-breaking work there, which showed that animals exposed to snake venom yielded an effective antitoxin, helped to lay the foundation for the science of immunology. Sewall had come to

Colorado because of an illness, not recognized as tuberculosis, and was given a medical degree by the University of Denver in 1889 in consideration of his academic record. When he realized that he had tuberculosis, he went to Saranac Lake and became Trudeau's first resident physician. He held the chair in physiology at the University of Denver's Department of Medicine until 1908. In 1916, he became president of the Association of American Physicians; yet with all his honors, he retained his humility. The executive faculty minutes for June 25, 1917, report his desire for a demotion of his academic status: "Dr. Sewall feels that the title lecturer is more consonant with the amount of work he feels he can do."

Sewall and Waring became good friends. The younger man liked the emphasis Sewall put on the importance of teaching and on exciting the student's curiosity; he also appreciated his outspokenness about things he thought should be condemned. They shared a love of books; Sewall has been termed the father of the Colorado Medical Library Association, which was formed in 1893. Sewall had a brilliant mind and an appealing whimsical streak, which would have drawn Waring, who shared the trait, closer to him. Waring called him "Sir Henry." It was a fortunate association for Waring, who may have missed his correspondence with the now-deceased Trudeau. Similarly, it was a happy association for Sewall, who was childless.

Waring held his position as instructor of medicine from 1914 until 1917, when the regents declared all positions in the teaching staff vacant in order to effect a complete reorganization of the faculty. In June 1917 Dean Meader recommended that the department consist of himself as professor of medicine and head of Department of Medicine, with Henry Sewall as associate professor. That year the United States entered World War I, which had broken out in Europe in 1914 and was taking a devastating toll. Waring, thirty-four, regretted deeply his inability to serve because of his health. He served on the Medical Advisory Board of the state recruiting service and was appointed a member of the Colorado governing committee of the Gorgas Memorial Institute of Tropical and Preventive Medicine (established in honor of William C. Gorgas, who became surgeon general of the U.S. Army in 1914).

About this time Waring began writing papers; he eventually produced seventy-seven, over fifty-four of them scientific. He respected the written word, collecting books and reprints of papers, and reading a great deal. Noted cardiologist Paul Dudley White has written, "The more one reads the better medical works of past generations, the more astonished one becomes, and the more humble, too, at what has been known and written and then forgotten." His thoughts duplicated those of Waring, who spent a lifetime reading the old as well as the new, with a dictionary at his elbow.

Waring's first published paper, "Progress in the Study of Diseases of the Chest," appeared in *Colorado Medicine* in 1917. From the beginning he demonstrated a clear writing style, a feel for phrasing. "Probably not more than 1 percent of pulmonary disease is non-tuberculous in nature," he wrote. The statement, erroneous in view of what is known today, reflected the accepted thinking of that time. According to Dr. Roger Mitchell, an authority on pulmonary diseases, "There was then a lack of knowledge of diseases, such as chronic bronchitis and emphysema, as well as fungus diseases of lungs, and congenital disorders in children and adults." Waring concluded, "Wonderful have been the developments in, and the revelations by roentgenography [x-ray]; valuable has been the new laboratory work; but transcending these in importance and of far-reaching significance is the Framingham experiment—the first real attempt at comprehensive community hygiene in the United States." He not only gave early recognition to the importance of the Framingham study but probably was influenced by it to start an innovative industrial medical program at the medical school two decades later.

His second paper, "Relation of Recent Epidemic of Respiratory Diseases in Denver to Pulmonary Tuberculosis," which he read before the Denver Medical Society in 1917, was a commentary on diets prescribed as treatment, as observed in 120 patients with pulmonary tuberculosis. "Kidney problems may develop from diet," he wrote. Some treatments called for up to twelve eggs a day, up to two quarts of milk, roast beef, and beef juice, which is hard on kidneys and may cause albuminuria. Yet when Waring was recovering after a complication of tuberculosis a few years after he wrote this paper, part of his diet included juice extracted from raw beef.

Waring's relationship with Bonney ended, and he began working with a second partner, Dr. Leonard M. Van Stone, who was another Harvard Medical School graduate. Four years younger than Waring, he had served as a captain in the British Royal Army Medical Corps from 1917 to 1919. It is not known exactly when Waring met him, but a form stated that they were associated in 1925. They probably did not join forces until the 1920s, because in 1919 Waring fell victim to influenza, which turned into pneumonia. The executive faculty minutes of the medical school for September 26, 1919, noted that he was granted a leave of absence "for one year because of ill health."

Drs. Van Stone and Waring had their first offices in the Metropolitan Building. For a few years Waring's offices were listed at an address in the Imperial Building, but according to his letterhead, he was back in the Metropolitan Building in January 1936. But that was far in the future. The year that now bears scrutiny is 1920.

5 *Courtship, Marriage and General Practice*

"YOU HAVE A CAREER ahead of you which the right woman will help, the wrong woman wreck," William Osler wrote to a young graduate. Osler had many things to say about marriage; another way he put it was, "Put your affections in cold storage for a few years, and you will take them out ripened—perhaps a bit mellow."

About the time James Waring was preparing to re-enter medical school, Trudeau had written, "You will be lonely, dear boy, without your friends. . . . Tell me, who do you see most of these days and what girl do you like?" But there does not seem to have been a woman in Waring's life since Edith Duer. Then, sometime early in 1920, at a small dinner party for four people, Waring met Ruth Porter. He would turn thirty-seven that year and she would turn thirty-one. Between May and August 1920 Waring was in California as part of a rest cure after la grippe the previous year had turned into pneumonia. He wrote to Ruth two or three times, and she answered.

Blue-eyed Ruth Porter was shy, or more accurately, reserved, brought up to put self-discipline, duty, orderliness, thriftiness, and correct behavior ahead of many other virtues. But she was not strait-laced. She had a good sense of humor and could be a comic with family and close friends, preferring small social gatherings to large ones. She had attended Miss Summers's School in Washington, D.C. (later Mount Vernon Seminary and today Mount Vernon College), was a member of the board of directors of Children's Hospital, and took part in such social groups as the Wednesday Music Party and the Little Theater. She also was building a house in Evergreen in the mountains west of Denver.

The Porter family had a considerable fortune, which might be called "quiet money." Ruth's father, Henry M. Porter, a successful entrepreneur, had retired three years previously at the age of seventy-nine. He had given his five children equal assets and devoted the rest of his long life giving to worthy causes and writing about his philosophical views. His philanthropies were fired by his belief, shared with Andrew Carnegie, that the man who dies rich dies disgraced.

Waring's dark eyes were his most notable feature, described as "the darkest, biggest, sparklingest eyes" or, as in the Yale yearbook, "black Southern eyes." Many have commented on how they twinkled. His mother also was noted for her dark eyes, and presumably his Basque father's eyes would have been dark, too. Although his eyes may have been described as "Southern," Waring did not speak with a southern accent after so many years spent away from the South. In assessing himself a few months later in a letter to Ruth, he wrote: "I am a quiet, reserved sort of chap—feeling deeply about serious things and prone not to talk much about things that lie near my heart. This reserve is partly natural and partly due to my long period of sickness during which I mingled very little socially."

With their mutual reserve and discipline, they might have taken months longer to get closer, despite their growing fondness for each other, had not Ruth been about to leave at the end of November. Every winter her father and mother went to California to be near their daughter Dora, known as Dodie, and her husband, John Thomas Mason, who lived in Pasadena. Ruth, the youngest of the five Porter children and the only one still unmarried, usually accompanied them, staying from December to May. She acted as part-time surrogate mother to a young niece, Laurene Walker, whose mother, Laurene Porter Walker (Ruth's sister), had died in 1916, and whose father, Harold Struther Walker, had died from influenza in the 1918 epidemic when she was seven.

"The thirties seem to be the fateful time for the Waring men," James's Aunt Martha (Uncle Pinck's wife) would later write to him, "and the lady going on a trip seems to bring things to a head; it was so in our case, and Pinck has been chuckling over the same thing happening in yours." Things did indeed come to a head, and rather quickly. How James's and Ruth's letters changed in late 1920! Although Ruth saved all of his, he saved only some of hers. On November 30, she wrote:

> Dearest Jim
> Just a wee note to say I am so happy that I am miserable. Have just put a letter in the box telling mother and father the glad tidings. Won't you please see them before they leave. They close the house Friday and leave Monday. I asked them to say nothing and said you would tell only your Mother.
> Love and kisses, Ruthie

On the same day, James wrote Ruth, saying that he would soon have a talk with her father and also with his mother:

> Shall heave a sigh of relief when I get both of these interviews off my chest. The more I think of it Ruthie, the more nerve I think I

> had to ask you to marry me, for I have so darn little to offer you and on the other hand there is so much you can do to help me in the present work I am doing and then to advance on further to finer things. . . . At this critical moment I find myself with my bank balance thoroughly depleted so I am starting to save for that ring first and will have it as quick as I can get the one I want for you. You see I am not a wealthy man, Ruthie. Nearly all I have I have earned myself by hard work. . . . My speed at best is not very great, Ruthie. I am counting on you for sympathy and understanding of this particular infirmity of mine. . . . Help me to go slowly and you will find that year by year I will be able to do more. Our great American dream anyhow is 'Speed' and we too frequently lose sight and touch of the finer things by so continually hustling. . . . I love you very dearly and with all my heart.

In a letter to James dated December 2, Ruth wrote:

> [It was] just a week ago tonight that you gathered up your courage and said the fatal words that have robbed you of your independence and freedom. I should hate myself to find that I had led you on to speak before you were ready. Jim do let us be honest with each other. . . . If you can and will answer me honestly and blot out the doubt I promise never to mention it or let it bother me again.

Replying to her doubts about his proposal, James wrote: "Now Ruthie! I wish I had you here right now that I might tell you again how much I care—and how good I will be to you and most of all how good I hope you will be to me."

Also in Ruth's letter of December 2 was this effort to ease his concerns about her wealth:

> Jim please don't worry about not being a wealthy man. The fact that you have gotten what you have by your own efforts means more to me than untold wealth. You have enough to make us happy and comfortable without considering what I have and wish I didn't or hadn't. . . . My unearned share of our material possessions I hope with your guidance to use wisely and to a great extent for those who are unfortunate and deserve more than they have.

As a medical student he had underlined in his Marcus Aurelius: "From my mother I learned . . . simplicity in my way of living, far removed from the habits of the rich." Her words may have helped assuage any doubts he may have had.

In an undated letter, James reported to Ruth on his discussion with his mother and his "interview" with the Porters:

> They all dealt gently with me. Mother is so devoted to me that her one great fear is that when I marry the unfortunate lady who draws me may not be nice to her. . . . She will meet you more than half way and I know you will be good to her, at first for my sake and later for her own.
>
> Your Father and Mother were very gentle with me. The old gentleman would digress to talk about "Judge Springer" and the Old Days while I sweated with nervousness. Then Will [Ruth's brother] and Mrs. [Permelia Curtis] Will arrived and while your mother was letting them in your father in a voice plainly audible in the hall by Will, I am sure, he said, "I take it, Doctor, that you have led a clean and pure life?" I trust he approved my emphatic "Yes, Sir." The worst I ever did was to dance with that red-headed delegate to the Democratic Convention in San Francisco and I never saw her before. For which, Mademoiselle, I crave your humble pardon! . . . Now Ruthie! I wish I had you here right now that I might tell you again how much I care—and how good I will be to you and most of all how good I hope you will be to me.

What he failed to mention was that when asking for Ruth's hand, James said to Henry Porter, "I've had tuberculosis"—to which the elderly gentleman replied that he had suffered it, too.

On December 5, James wrote to Ruth: "I have had a very slight return of the same symptoms I had in California and the question arises whether I should not have my appendix out. (This would be a recurring topic in coming weeks. Waring eventually obtained a third opinion about his health from his friend, Henry Sewall. After checking his lungs and his appendix, reported the patient, "He said I could get life insurance on the soundness of the former and all thought of operation for appendicity in his opinion was bunk!")

The same day, she replied: "When I think of becoming Mrs. Waring, the wife of a man who has made a name for himself in this relentless world and against such great odds, it just plain scares me and makes me wonder how you can really care. You have done so much and I so little!"

On December 7, he wrote:

> Mother loved your letter and so did I. I am so glad you wrote her. My best girl friend I have had [presumably Edith Duer] she always approved of, but she says a man's judgment in affairs of the heart is never to be relied upon. . . . Even now I can scarcely believe all the happiness [that] is coming to me. Don't worry. I shall play a little—that is I shan't work too hard.
>
> For twenty years I have had darn little in the way of fun and very little more in the shape of real happiness. Spartan discipline nearly all the time and the rest of it hard work and still more hard work. So I should not really be very hard to make happy or keep happy.

On Sunday, December 12, he wrote a long letter in response to Ruth's plea for a "personal history."

> Sunday morning—gentle snowstorm and I am bundled up on my sleeping porch writing you. . . . I was born August 11, 1883 in Savannah, Ga.—of the usual poor but honest parents. Very early in my youth—I was about 18 months old—my father proved himself a slacker, so Mother promptly got a divorce with custody of my brother and myself.

It was a long letter, giving the rest of the major details of his life, and ended, "Love me much and all the time and we will have the happiest home in Denver! There will be none any happier. I know that!" So there it was, out in the open, although he omitted his father's name. Now, with his past revealed, a lightheartedness slipped into his writing, except for his continuing concern about his health. In one letter he compared himself to "the Mississippi River steamboat that had just enough steam pressure in its boilers to whistle or paddle, it couldn't paddle and whistle at the same time."

A few days after writing the "personal history" letter, Waring bought an engagement ring at Bohm-Allen in Denver and had it sent to California—Ruth and Laurene were staying in La Jolla—by special delivery. The postman delivered the package in the early evening, and Ruth, seeing him coming, ran out to the sidewalk to receive it. She then stood there, opening the box, and somehow, in her excitement, dropped the ring. In the deepening twilight, she and the kindly postman spent some twenty minutes searching on their hands and knees, joined by occasional passers-by. Fortunately, the ring was found and never again strayed from Ruth's possession until she gave it to her grandson, Edward D. White III, when he became engaged.

In his next letter, James expressed many feelings and thoughts more openly than ever before:

> I have had more of real happiness in the past ten days since our memorable Sunday night than in all the rest of my life put together. An entirely new and wonderful existence has been unfolding itself in my thoughts. I have been making plans and "wildly speculating." Also! Have no doubt of me or my affection. I'm a square guy and could never ask any girl to marry me unless I cared and had a good hunch she cared. I confess to being a coward in this matter Ruthie—timid of whether I could make you happy since I am not strong. Don't think it childish for in spite of it I have been very reckless of my health and strength. You will understand then this fear of mine and my desire that I should physically be able to keep up with you in your activities wherever they might lead us.
>
> If you really care deeply for me, you will be happy with me because my limited strength will keep me near the home fire side and make our existence a close one. I am a home builder and a home lover. Every nickel and penny I own is as sweet and clean as you could wish it and the thought back of that has been because I don't want anything to come near me or my home that isn't sweet and clean.
>
> I have as I said had darn little real happiness in this life so far. Since I was 24 I have been more or less disabled—utterly deprived of all that you and I call fun. . . . You can help me not only to be a good doctor, not only in treating the sick, perhaps later in public health work, perhaps in research work, but also in putting into my life that real joy in your affection and comradeship that without you I would not have.

He reiterated his plan to rest in Santa Fe from January to April, work hard in May and June, marry in July, and "go at once anywhere you say—just so there's no hay fever there." As for their future residence, he wanted "a modest mansion out of the smoky district, with a view of the mountains." He was glad she wanted a quiet wedding and said he would not give a stag dinner: "They are orgies."

In his next letter, the groom-to-be talked about Hilltop, Ruth's new house in Evergreen, and his fear of hay fever there. "I am afraid of the frightful paroxysms of sneezing which threaten to tear loose my adhesions in my chest. This means that July and August for the next year or two will be my big cautious time." He was also worried about his appendix again and said he could not come to Pasadena for Christmas because he might need an operation, even though three doctors had assured him he did not.

Their letters of December 18 crossed. Ruth wrote: "It is like being freed from prison to be out of that artificial atmosphere of Pasadena. You don't know how I long every waking moment to be with you. . . . Why I should deserve such a true and deep happiness is absolutely a mystery to me." She wanted to see Laurene through the school term in La Jolla, where she attended Miss Bishop's School as a day student. She thought a family wedding was a good idea; she could not see herself in a white wedding dress but would like to be married in a small church.

They discussed Laurene's future. Ruth wrote that if they took her niece to live in her house on Logan Street it would be hard "with memories of Laurene and Harold [the girl's parents]." Jim wrote: "Laurene must come to live with us—we, at least I can't go to live with her in her family's home." Writing on December 21, Waring took in good humor Jack Mason's remark about his being bald and said he could not have his picture taken until he had a haircut, adding, "Tell Jack what I say—he will be amused!" He tacked on a P.S.: "Christmas always gives me a terrible heartache for a wife—kiddies and my own fireside."

Christmas passed with telegrams and the kind of presents considered proper between unmarried people: a scarf for him, candy, books, and flowers for her. On the day after Christmas he wrote: "I didn't go to church—rarely do go although I have a deep religious faith that has left me saying my prayers with great regularity for now some 30 odd years or more. Sunday is my day of rest and it helps me marvellously just to loaf around the house. When I go, I usually go on the first Sunday in the month."

On January 3, 1921, he told of missing lawyer and poet James Grafton Rogers's tea and muffin party at the Cactus Club. "In the programme this week is the Twelfth Night celebration at the University Club." On the same day Ruth wrote: "If you don't hear from me for a few weeks you'll know I'm deep in the throes of writing up my account book from the 1st of Jan. 1920." (This remained a habit of Ruth's through the years; it was her brother Will, reportedly, who suggested she get into the habit of keeping her account books herself.) The next day she wrote: "If I let you buy the lots for our home will you let me build the house or at least help. I am crazy to make the floor plans and have Jacques [Benedict, a well-known architect] do the elevation but want to know what type of house appeals to you. I don't want anything large or elaborate but well arranged and good. . . . Shall it be Colonial, English, plain American stucco or what?"

Their friends were becoming inquisitive about their unannounced engagement, but the couple did not want an announcement until their plans had been set. Ruth's missing letters must have included pleas that he come to California, because his letters of early January expressed anxiety regarding his health and showed a tinge of annoyance that she did not understand its precariousness. In a letter of January 4 he told her of his prudent regime: "In bed nearly every night at 7 o'clock—weekends quietly resting at home, no thought of trips into the mountains, no dances and only rarely a dinner party." He told at length the sacrifices that would have to be made on account of his physical disability, exclaiming, "Ah! Ruthie, am I asking too much?" Poor Ruth, engaged but alone, with little company except that of her niece and her parents, would not take no for an answer to her entreaties that he come to La Jolla. James's next letter, January 7, went over the same ground:

> I certainly jumped when I saw that you had me arriving on a train at La Jolla. If you try to bust up my medical career this way, Young Lady, I see where you'll be paying for our board and keep before the honeymoon is well over. . . . All during September and October when I was refusing invitations to spend the weekend at Evergreen and Hilltop I was spending from Saturday noon to Monday a.m. in bed on my porch and taking all my meals in bed. . . . Two years--no! even one year of the wrong kind of married life and you would have an invalid husband on your hands—my Pride in the dust and my heart broken.

After Ruth received this letter, the question of an immediate reunion was shelved—for a while.

Fewer of Ruth's letters survive than of his. Hers show a happy young woman in love. She was sympathetic with her fiancé's woes and reluctant to mention any of her own. In one letter she mentions a "fiendish sick headache—will call the doctor if it isn't better. Please don't think me a grumbler. I will buck up and not mention my trifling troubles again." He, on the other hand, would occasionally grumble. "Have had a hard day by which I mean lots of work. My sick people—

much anxiety and considerable querulousness to contend with. Curious how people demand so much consideration from the Doctor and give him so d— little."

They continued to discuss house plans. Again James's health came up, and he wrote that a complete x-ray of his gastrointestinal tract had revealed no ulcer, no gallstones, and no tuberculosis. The x-ray physician thought appendicitis possible, but the evidence was not sufficient to justify an operation.

A letter of January 24 announced his coming to La Jolla in mid-February. He would stay with Ruth's brother, John Porter (married to Louise Coors), for proper chaperonage. He liked the house plans she had sent him. On January 25 he told her he wanted to marry her "because I thought you cared and because I did . . . because I thought you were also a sweetly reasonable woman who would forgive and help me with my physical limitations . . . because of what I may call your interest in sick people and sympathy for them. A Doctor's wife has to have a great love of suffering humanity at large and in general, but also in particular."

His mood was far different a few days later: "You mustn't mind the sober tone of my letter. I pass through periods of depression every bit of which is due to fatigue and anxiety about my work and also largely to the constant exhausting effort of putting fight into people who would quit fighting if you didn't make them. The constant effort to keep others cheerful after a while gets to be a damn bore and believe me I get fed up on sick people (including myself) once in a while." But he was cheerful two days later and told of taking "Rob Stearns and wife to a little supper at the Country Club last night." On February 11, apparently discussing where and when to get married, he wrote: "Any time—anywhere with Mother present or it surely would break her heart to have me slip off without her being present and indeed I wouldn't feel as if I were properly married without her blessing!"

By then, the news of their engagement had finally leaked. A letter of January 28 to Ruth states: "Well, the fat is in the fire! I would guess the 'news' is over the town now." It literally was all over town by early February. "Society will be particularly interested in the betrothal of Miss Ruth Porter," began the article in the *Rocky Mountain News* society column. "Miss Porter, who occupies a prominent position in exclusive Denver society, is sojourning in La Jolla, California, with her parents at present. She is unusually charming and clever and takes an active part in the social life of Denver. . . . Dr. Waring will depart Wednesday for the coast."

Here the packet of letters comes to an end; the engaged pair were together, fully chaperoned, from February on. Once more, Waring's health forced him to alter his plans: On the day they originally had chosen for their wedding, he had his appendix out. For that reason, the wedding—finally held on June 15, 1921—was very quiet, with only the family and a few close friends present in St. Martin's Chapel of St. John's Cathedral, Denver. They honeymooned at Hilltop, which was a mile from Troutdale, a resort above Evergreen. The land had been given to Ruth by her father, and she had her house built on a hill looking toward the mountain range to the west, dominated by Mount Evans, and down on the beautiful Bendemere Valley. As planned, the house, built of granite, was designed by architect Jacques Benedict.

Then they settled into a rented house in the city while going over plans with Benedict for the house in Denver each had long dreamed of. Among Waring's mementos is a pocket notebook with a card from Ruth: "A wee gift in memory of November 28, 1920. This little bird echoes the song that has been constantly in my heart since that happy day." They were on their way to a stable and enduring marriage. James Waring, as it turned out, had followed his mentor, Osler, to the letter: "One of the most important lessons to be gathered . . . is—marry the right woman." A friend of both James Waring and Ruth Porter says they were very "unalike" but that it was a very happy marriage.

Ruth Porter Waring was seen as reserved, even distant, by people who knew her only casually. According to family members, she had difficulty meeting new people. Perhaps being the youngest of five children and taught to give precedence to age left her with a tendency to be quiet, a "private" person. Close friends spoke of her warmth, her willingness to listen to their problems, her sense of fun. Clearly, though, socializing did not come naturally to her. When Ruth attended Miss Summers's School in Washington, D.C., she once was locked out of her room so that she "would be more sociable." She accepted this as a necessary part of her "education." In the same way, though young and unmarried, she accepted her assignment when asked by her parents to help bring up Laurene Porter Walker.

In order to understand Ruth better, it would help to take a look at her family, which brought together two of Denver's pioneer families. At the time Ruth and James met, she was living at home with her parents in a twenty-room red brick house at 975 Grant Street on Capitol Hill in Denver. Henry Porter had had the house built in 1913 by architect Maurice Biscoe. Despite its size, it was lacking in the ostentation of the more ornate mansions of the era; it was solid, with few embellishments, though it had a lovely south-facing walled garden and a trellised walkway. The Porters did not want to attract attention to themselves.[17]

Henry Miller Porter, born in 1838 in Lancaster, Pennsylvania, had known severe privation as a child, his family moving from one frontier farm to another, each one farther west. At one time, John Benjamin Porter, his wife, Henrietta, and their daughter and three sons lived in a one-room log cabin with two beds and a trundle bed. At twenty, Henry Porter got a job as a laborer with the Stebbins Telegraph Company of Atchison, Kansas, and laid a section of the transcontinental line. At age twenty-four he became a partner of his employer, Charles M. Stebbins. They next freighted goods from Atchison to Denver in 1862. Showing vision and enterprise, by 1864 he was organizing wagon trains to supply gold fields in the West. He became involved in building and later in financing railroads, including the Denver Pacific Railroad line to Cheyenne.

Always diversifying, he turned to cattle ranching in New Mexico during the 1870s, eventually running 60,000 head and controlling two million acres of grazing land. In 1873 he became the president of the first independent telegraph company in Colorado, the United States and Mexico Telegraph Company. Five years later he became president of the first telephone company in New Mexico.

Porter did not put down roots in Denver until he returned there in 1883. As he became involved in business in Denver, he continued to manage his ranching interests and to develop real estate holdings in ten western states. Charitable enterprises began to occupy more of his efforts: he was a founder and director of the Denver Museum of Natural History (he would serve on the board of trustees for thirty-seven years) and he extensively aided various educational and philanthropic organizations. Porter was among the many leading citizens in the Colorado Forestry and Horticultural Association, formed in 1884, one of the first forestry associations established in the United States.[18]

It is tempting to attribute Porter's philanthropy, much of it anonymous, to his upbringing, for his maternal grandfather was a German Lutheran minister. Although considered a nominal Episcopalian, Porter did not attend church. Still, he considered Sunday a day of rest, with no card playing allowed in his home. He was described as living "a scrupulously careful life," with "none of the habits and vices which discount the quality and cut short the longevity of so many men today." The Porter children learned the value of commitment to the community, of sharing and of using talents to help others without expecting praise and accolades.

Because Porter was a larger-than-life figure, his wife's family is overshadowed. Laura Porter's father, John W. Smith, also was born in Pennsylvania. Showing the same enterprising spirit as his future son-in-law, Smith brought a wagon train containing machinery from Kansas into Denver in 1860. Later he built various mills and a hotel, started a cracker factory, and became a railroad president. One of the less utilitarian things he brought to Denver was a melodeon, which is still in the family's possession today.

Smith is best remembered for "Smith's Ditch," also known as the "City Ditch" or the "Big Ditch." He took an unproductive ditch company in the mid-1860s and built a new channel with a sufficient grade to bring water from the South Platte to Denver. The new aqueduct helped bring trees, lawns, and gardens to the city on the plains. Smith's Ditch still provides water for both lakes at Denver's Washington Park and flows into City Park Lake. Some segments of City Ditch still flow above ground in Washington Park.

This was Ruth Porter Waring's heritage, unlike her husband's in many ways, yet they had much in common. They both had experienced prolonged residence with their families. Because of his illness, Waring had stayed with his mother for years. Although she dated, went to parties, and loved to dance, Ruth Porter was still bound by the routine of going with her parents and her niece to California for five months of every year. When they married, they must have gained a sense of freedom from the loving but binding ties of their relatives.

When it came to picking an architect for their house in Denver they turned, naturally, to Jules Jacques Benois Benedict, who had designed Hilltop.[19] The site of the house-to-be was on East Ninth Avenue at Gaylord Street in Morgan's Subdivision. It was on high ground, south of what today is the Denver Botanic Gardens but then was called Mount Calvary, maintained as a cemetery by the Catholic church. Ruth was pregnant at the time the house was being built. It was supposed to be ready for occupancy by Christmas 1922, but the couple may have been at the Porters' house at 975 Grant Street at the time of the birth of their daughter, Ruth Porter, on February 25, 1923. Accounts vary as to their whereabouts at this time.

The stresses of having a house built, expecting his first child, and running his practice may have taken their toll on James Waring. After his bout with pneumonia in 1919 and his appendectomy just before his wedding in 1921, the doctor's next bout of illness came in late 1922, when Ruth was in the late stages of her pregnancy with Ruth. James went to Baltimore for a complete checkup and while there he called

Mrs. Douglas Duer, the mother of his old girlfriend Edith. Mrs. Duer sent a car and chauffeur to bring him to stay with her and take him wherever he wanted to go. His illness was diagnosed as colitis, with no serious organic disease and no tuberculosis. He was put on belladonna drops, a diet stressing fruits and vegetables, emulsions of olive oil, and "plenty of rest and don't worry."

He need not have worried about the house: Benedict did not disappoint the Warings. The house he designed eventually would achieve landmark status, along with others of his design in the city. It was stucco, painted a soft sage green, accented with stonework and crowned with a roof of green tiles. This was not the "small but comfortable house" the Warings had first envisioned; it was one of a series of stunning homes the celebrated architect was designing for Denver's best neighborhoods. The interior of 910 Gaylord, in particular, showed his loving attention, with Ruth's close collaboration. After entering the wide front hall, a visitor would see, to the right, a spacious living room, used mostly for parties, though the couple did not entertain often. Allen Tupper True, a renowned Denver artist, had decorated the mantelpiece with flowers, butterflies, rabbits, centaurs, and lightly clad maidens ("non-sexy ladies" and "remarkably unsensual" are family assessments of them today), adding a bit of lightness and frivolity to the decor. When a later occupant's decorator disliked the mural over the fireplace, it was painted over in the 1950s, to the sorrow of the Warings.

On the advice of decorator Thornton Fuller, the wood furniture was covered in dark burgundy and green tapestry and brocade. The walls were sand-colored and rough in texture. The carpets were rich, dark Orientals, and heavy draperies at the windows reduced the light from outside. At the garden end of the room were two windows and eventually two grand pianos, lighted by the handsome arched portals. What made the living room so special was True's Italianate decoration of the ceiling, dispelling any heaviness in the room's decor. The gifted artist, whose murals were commissioned for the rotunda walls of the Colorado State Capitol, the walls of the original Colorado National Bank Building, and the Brown Palace Hotel lobby, was equally talented in designing residential decor. That which he created for 910 Gaylord Street artfully complements the intricate terra-cotta and stone doorways and window lintels and the graceful stairways of Jacques Benedict.

Adjoining the living room was a small, cheerful sunroom-library where Ruth retreated every morning to her orderly desk, keeping her meticulous accounts. Beyond this room, at the end of the hall, were the dining room, pantry, kitchen, a small servants' dining room, and, curiously, a phone booth. Outside, again under Ruth's careful supervision, the landscaping provided needed shade in Denver's hot summers, and borders of flowers set off the house with splashes of color. A big Russian olive tree in the garden had a bench at its base, all in a large well-tended garden enclosed by wrought-iron fencing.

A handsome winding staircase led to the second floor, where the Warings slept in a glass-enclosed sleeping porch on the south side of the house. In summer the windows were opened and screens were put in place. This was an early-to-bed household. Waring usually came home for lunch and had a rest before returning to the office or classroom. When he came home in the afternoon, he would usually lie down and have another rest before dinner, sometimes bundling up and falling asleep in the big chair on the downstairs porch. Then he would spend a few hours after dinner reading and studying in bed, wearing a green eyeshade. His regimen was not out of the ordinary for that era. Dr. Fred Ayvazian, in "The Fifty-five Trudeau Medalists," wrote, "Having reached a true recovery—a tolerable adjustment—many long-term 'lungers'—no matter how actively employed they became, or symptom-free they remained, they retained habits of daily rest hours, early bedtimes, strict schedules of annual X rays." So it was with James Waring.

A second daughter, Anne Johnston, was born to the Warings on April 7, 1924. Not long after Anne's birth, Waring's mother wrote to Antonio, "Do teach your children to kiss and be kissed on the cheek." She would never be able to pass along this advice to her other son. Although James sometimes hugged his daughters, his kisses were always carefully placed on the backs of their necks for fear of infecting them with tuberculosis.

The Warings' house had been built with children in mind. A pleasant, sunny nursery, where the girls usually had their meals, stood at the head of the stairs; it later served as Anne's bedroom until she was a teenager. Ruth had an adjoining room, and they shared a bathroom, which had the unusual feature of a separate basin for toothbrushing, a feature insisted upon by their father, ever mindful of tuberculosis and its germs. This floor also included a guest room, with a spectacular mountain view to the west; a large but cozy upstairs sitting room, which also contained a bed and chairs; a room for Laurene; and two small bedrooms near the back stair. On the third floor was an unfinished attic space that Waring eventually had made into a large library-study, with stacks to house his ever-growing book collection. The third floor also had a small playroom.

As much as Ruth loved her husband and children, she needed

respite from the confines of motherhood, judging by the trips she took on her own when the girls were infants. In February 1925, six months after Anne's birth, she went to the Coronado Hotel to join her parents and Laurene, leaving the babies with their father and a nursemaid. In May she went to a reunion of Mount Vernon Seminary (it may still have been called Miss Summers's School then) in Washington, D.C. In September, when she went to New York, Waring was lonely, showing anxiety in his letters. When making plans to attend a medical meeting, he wrote that he did not like to leave the babies when she was away and that he could "hardly sleep thinking about them and nearly gave up my trip I was so unhappy." He traveled, too, going to medical meetings and on fishing trips, and he joined Ruth in bringing Laurene, who always needed a chaperon for her travels, home from some connecting point, occasionally accompanied by her classmates.

When the Porters built a new house at Ninth and Vine Streets, a couple of blocks away from 910 Gaylord Street, Ruth may have felt increased parental demands upon her. After Ruth and James were newly married, Houstoun Waring arrived in Colorado; his father was George Waring, a cousin of Annie. Houstoun (pronounced "House-ton" and called "Hous" by friends and family) Waring had contracted tuberculosis while attending Naval Academy and in 1921 was sent to Fort Lyon Tuberculosis Hospital for the Navy, near Las Animas, Colorado. Later in the year naval officers were shipped to Fitzsimons Hospital east of Denver, and in 1922 he went to stay with the Warings for a week or two. He settled in Colorado, eventually becoming editor of the *Littleton Independent.*

According to Houstoun, his cousin sent a dozen roses to Ruth "every Saturday after they were married." For how long, he does not say, but the reminiscence confirms Waring's devotion. And so began a marriage, husband and wife happily sharing what gifts they had and developing enduring respect and affection for each other. As Waring wrote his wife on December 10, 1925: "The peace and sanctity of 910 Gaylord Street is what I love and that means you—for you make the home!!"

In the mid-1920s James Waring had a busy general practice with Leonard Van Stone and was interested in learning about many diseases that came under the heading of "internal medicine." Although he may never have intended to become an expert in tuberculosis, according to Houstoun Waring, he acquired that reputation. Waring was one of the first experts in the disease who was not directly associated with a sanatorium.

When asked to serve as assistant professor of medicine at the University of Colorado School of Medicine, he gladly accepted. The year was 1926, and it followed a year of great changes at the medical school. In January 1925 the new medical center was opened on Colorado Boulevard and East Ninth Avenue, with classrooms; a 150-bed hospital, Colorado General, that could be expanded to 300 beds; a psychopathic hospital; nurses' quarters; and a power plant. Archer House, the old rented house where the junior and senior years of medical school had long been taught, was woefully inadequate, and the need for a state-controlled general hospital for teaching purposes was apparent. Thanks to a grant of $700,000 from the General Education Board of the Rockefeller Foundation in 1922, the medical school could proceed with plans for construction, providing that the state of Colorado raised a matching amount–and match it the state did.

It was a time of change, too, within the Department of Medicine. Since 1916, Charles N. Meader, M.D., had served as professor of medicine and as dean of the medical school. He resigned as dean in July 1925 and was succeeded by Dr. Maurice Rees. Also in 1925 Dr. Franklin Ebaugh became the first official full-time clinical faculty member, appointed director of the psychopathic hospital and professor of psychiatry on a twelve-month basis. The concept of a salary for full-time faculty members would prove to be controversial. When Waring became assistant professor, his work for the medical school, like that of his colleagues, was unpaid. Others in the Department of Medicine included Drs. Rudolph W. Arndt, Constantine F. Kemper, and C. T. Burnett. Like most doctors in private practice, Waring had regular sessions in his office to take care of before he could leave for the medical school to teach.

Other changes were also under way. Since its beginning, Colorado General Hospital had been thought of in the community as a place for the indigent to receive treatment. No patient ever would be refused treatment because of inability to meet the specified charges, according to the state legislature's actions of 1921. However, some patients were asked to pay for some or all of the per diem hospital charge. At the December 7, 1925, meeting of the Executive Faculty Committee, it was moved and approved that the "matter of free patients be left entirely to the discretion of the superintendent of the hospital." The issue remained a thorny one.

During this period, James Waring discovered another passion: teaching. He began to distinguish himself at grand rounds, the meeting of the general faculty held one evening a month in the clinical amphitheater. Grand rounds were teaching exercises given for the benefit of students and residents by the faculty members involved in patient care. Waring discussed an extraordinary range of topics: kidney function, lung abscess and bronchiectasis complicating diabetes mellitus, closed drainage of empyema, gunshot wound of the chest with complications, aortic aneurysm and syphilis, Hodgkin's disease, and a new method of treating snakebite.

Waring enjoyed young people. He went out of his way to help them and took a great interest in their careers, giving a boost when he could. When Alpha Omega Alpha, a medical honor society, established a chapter at the University of Colorado in 1926, he became actively involved and was given an honorary membership that year. His relationship with the society remained close through the years; members knew they could count on his support when it was needed.

One student of this period stood out in particular: Ward Darley, a 1929 graduate who had a residency at Colorado General Hospital. He later would become dean of the medical school and eventually president of the University of Colorado. In a letter to Paul Anderson, a student in 1963 who wrote a biography of Waring, Darley recalled that Waring "was a superb teacher who . . . had more of an impact on me than any physician I could name. His influence was particularly important during my residency. In those days there was only one resident in medicine and, as a consequence, I pretty much received his full attention." Another outstanding student of this period was Dr. Abe Ravin, class of 1932, who later came to be known as the first full-time cardiologist west of the Mississippi River.

Waring's devotion to teaching did not keep him from continuing to publish occasional writings. Between 1922 and 1929, he produced three papers on roentgenography, or x-rays, in collaboration with W. Walter Wasson, M.D. His work with Dr. Wasson in Denver helped to establish improved x-ray techniques for chest examinations. The proper interpretation of the roentgenogram, Waring believed, depended upon the use of two procedures: auscultation, or listening to the chest through a stethoscope; and percussion, or tapping the chest wall with a finger to bring out differences in the density of the lung. Through the years he emphatically stressed the importance of these techniques to his medical students.

In "Relapse in Pulmonary Tuberculosis" (1923), Waring wrote that for the victim of tuberculosis "the sudden strain of cranking an automobile may prove as harmful as the prolonged overexertion of heavy manual labor. The former acts by tearing open an old lesion in pleura or lung, the latter usually by its accumulated depression of vital forces. . . . Overplay is more dangerous than overwork." These words would haunt him eight years later.

In "Tobacco and Tuberculosis" (1924), Waring reached conclusions on the health hazards of smoking that showed him to be far ahead of his time. The surgeon general's report on the effects of smoking would not be published for another forty years; scientists needed decades to prove beyond doubt that cigarettes cause cancer and heart disease. Arthur M. Olsen, M.D., former chairman of the subdivision on pulmonary disease of the American Board of Internal Medicine, wrote: "In my early days at Mayo Clinic . . . chest physicians and surgeons began to advise their patients to stop smoking." He was referring to 1938, fourteen years after Waring's paper was published.

Waring quoted studies that showed that "smoking increases expectoration and commonly aggravates a preexisting cough; smoking increases lassitude; smoking not infrequently causes a rise in temperature." Smoking, he noted, also can raise the blood pressure, increase pulse rate and cause a lack of appetite. All of the above, he explained, are particularly damaging to tuberculosis patients. "The prevailing opinion appears to be that the tuberculous patient is better off without tobacco, but the responsibility for decision is frequently passed to the patient himself. The average American resents prohibition. . . . Doctors prefer moral suasion to an attempt at military discipline with its inevitable evasion."

In a follow-up article, published in *Hygeia* in June 1925, Waring laid down rules for the smoker: "Do not smoke until past the age of twenty-one years"; "Do not inhale and blow smoke through the nose"; "Smoke outdoors and never indoors"; and, "At least once a year stop smoking for a month or more." Both papers on tobacco demonstrate a curious ambivalence. Waring's empathy with the smoker was apparent, as when he stated, in "Tobacco and Tuberculosis," "Sometimes, the patient himself is a smoker and skeptic as to the harmfulness of tobacco," adding, "The physician simply hates to be disagreeable about the matter; he knows that tobacco is a real solace in the irksomeness of prolonged 'Chasing the Cure.'"

Paradoxically, he had taken up smoking sometime in his life, perhaps at Yale or Hopkins—exactly when is not known. Some of his mentors smoked: William Welch smoked five cigars at the Nu Sigma Nu meeting Waring described in a letter to his mother. In his biography of Henry Sewall, Gerald Webb relates that when Sewall returned to Wesleyan in the fall of 1873 with a meerschaum pipe, several of his fellow students lectured him on the wickedness of his ways. He wrote and asked his mother's permission. She gave him the pipe, with some cigars thrown in for good measure. Osler smoked and so did his students, when they were guests at his house, having "'baccy and beer." Waring fought the habit, using chewing gum as a substitute for smoking during the early 1920s. Ruth teased him about the gum-chewing habit. Daughter Anne recalls that one day in the 1940s, when attending a dinner, he became dizzy and sick, later attributing this spell to smoking. Thereafter he gave up the habit.

In 1925 Waring wrote about the climate of Denver, explaining why it was regarded as beneficial for consumptives: "Denver has 302 annual days of sunshine, low humidity, and an altitude of 5,280 feet. The altitude causes deeper breathing and thus more red cells and hemoglobin. Dry, cool, moving air is best for lung patients." His statement that deeper breathing results in more red cells was later disproved. The increase in red cells associated with altitude is not, in fact, due to deep breathing but rather a response of the body that enables more oxygen to be carried in the blood. This knowledge was tucked away in a French medical journal in 1890, based on observations made on the natives of the high plains of South America.

A paper on hay fever in the Denver area, published in 1925, and one on the cotton of the cottonwood tree were of personal interest to Waring, a sufferer from the effects of pollens. He started a collection of literature on hay fever, which he later donated to the Denver Botanic Gardens library. A small greenhouse was built at 910 Gaylord where plants were raised for pollen studies. Waring's interest in allergies stemmed, in part, from a fear of prolonged sneezing, which he believed could tear adhesions in the chest, allowing the tubercle bacilli to reinfect and possibly causing a hemorrhage.

Some of Waring's writings focused on medical history. In "Villemin and the Transmissibility of Tuberculosis" (1926), Waring told of the debt owed by all physicians to Laënnec, inventor of the stethoscope, and questioned whether many "realize their debt to Villemin, who first proved the communicability of tuberculosis." Not surprisingly, Waring was chairman of the Laënnec Committee of the Denver Clinical and Pathological Society, which arranged a dinner commemorating the death of René Théophile Hyacinthe Laënnec. In February 1926 one hundred members and their guests gathered at the University Club and stood in tribute to Henry Sewall, who was ill, before James Waring delivered Sewall's address for him: "The Influence of [Pierre] Louis on American Medicine." At the end, two slides were shown of William Osler. In his account of the dinner in *Colorado Medicine,* Waring wrote: "With the last picture still on the screen and the closing lines of Sewall's paper in their ears: 'And Osler laid their wreath on the steps; and there we lay ours, too,' the hundred diners rose from their seats and stood for a few moments in silent tribute to Laënnec and Louis!"

Waring's own medical history brought him into contact, as both patient and colleague, with another physician who shared his devotion to medical history. One of his doctors from the Cragmor Sanitarium in Colorado Springs, Gerald Webb, had gone abroad in 1906, working several months in the laboratory of Almroth Wright, a renowned bacteriologist, at St. Mary's Hospital in London. His work there centered on immunity studies of "opsonins" (later to be called antibodies), from which Wright developed an "opsonic index," believing that one's immunity depended upon the amount of opsonin in his blood. After his return to the United States, Webb was in great demand as a speaker because of his familiarity with Wright's difficult new methods. Few in Colorado Springs shared his interest in research, however, and he was forced to do his experiments first in the garage in back of his house and later in space donated by Colorado College, financing most of his studies out of his own pocket and with a grant from the American Medical Association.

Webb had set an ambitious goal: the development of a vaccine to induce immunity to tuberculosis. One obstacle to finding a cure for tuberculosis comes from the waxlike coating that envelops the tubercle bacillus; the white corpuscles, which can devour organisms that cause many diseases, have difficulty digesting this waxy coating. Webb achieved his lasting fame by being the first in this country to recognize the importance of lymphocytes, one type of white corpuscle, in the process of immunity. He believed that this cell, which contains an enzyme known as lipase, which digests fats and wax, might fight the tubercle bacilli. Webb carried out lymphocyte experiments, hoping to destroy the waxy capsule. He also studied the effect of altitude on the lymphocyte count. For seven years Webb carried out these experiments, meeting defeat after defeat and eventually abandoning them. (It would be the mid-1970s before Webb's belief in the defensive role of lymphocytes would be vindicated.)

Webb became the first president of the newly founded American Association of Immunologists in 1913. Immunology was a new science, beginning in part with Henry Sewall's work with snake venom, and it provided a connecting link between Sewall and Webb, who possibly influenced Jim Waring more than any other physicians in Colorado.

Although both men were older (Sewall by twenty-eight years, Webb by twelve) and more research-minded than Waring, all three shared an interest in fighting tuberculosis, and all were scholars.

In 1920 Webb established the Colorado School for Tuberculosis, based on the theories of Trudeau's school in Saranac Lake. In furthering his research he enlisted the aid of Dr. William F. Drea, a dentist and radiologist in Colorado Springs, who was able to help by working in the laboratory on weekends and evenings. In 1923 they were joined by Dr. Charles Boissevain, a Dutchman who had contracted tuberculosis four years earlier. Working first in a small room in Palmer Hall on the Colorado College campus, they graduated to larger quarters four years later.

On May 15, 1924, the Colorado Foundation for Research in Tuberculosis was established as a nonprofit organization working to prevent and eventually to cure tuberculosis. Although the tubercle bacillus had been identified for over forty years, it had completely resisted all the conventional antitoxins and vaccines. James Waring was named one of four associate research directors, beginning a commitment which he would maintain through the years. The foundation took as its motto words from Descartes' *Discours de la Methode* (1637): Fac et Spera—Work and Hope.

Part Three | *Making His Mark*

6 *Thwarted Advocate*

JAMES WARING saw a need for a state tuberculosis hospital. In 1924 he was listed as "visiting physician" on the hospital service of Colorado General. The city tuberculosis dispensary was located in the Outpatient Department, where teaching in tuberculosis was conducted; Waring saw patients there whom he believed should be isolated in a sanatorium. Denver's population then was about 300,000 and Colorado's about one million.

In the January 1926 meeting of the Medical School and Hospital Development Committee, Waring presented a proposal to locate a tuberculosis sanatorium on the grounds of the new Colorado General Hospital. The seventeen-acre parcel of land given by Frederick Bonfils of *The Denver Post* allowed space for more buildings. The sanatorium was to be constructed in the near future under the auspices of the Denver Tuberculosis Society, the Denver Health Council, the Children's Hospital, and the Chamber of Commerce. Dean Maurice Rees read to the committee a letter from President Norlin indicating that the regents of the university had already shown approval in general terms. The committee approved the proposal. (These proceedings were recorded in the Executive Faculty Committee minutes of February 1, 1926.)

But something happened to scuttle the sanatorium initiative; Waring did not discuss it at the next Executive Faculty Committee meeting, nor is there another inclusion of the committee's reports among the Executive Faculty minutes. In March 1926 Waring resigned from the Medical School and Hospital Development Committee: "As president of the Denver Public Health Council I feel it most important that I should maintain as near as possible a non-partisan position about a number of the public health problems that concern us all."

The following year, however, Waring included an appeal for such a hospital in a talk on "Tuberculosis Control in Colorado." Speaking to the Colorado Conference of Social Workers, he pointed out that "Boulder County Hospital is the only county hospital besides the Denver General which has a ward for tuberculosis." He chastised the state and municipal health departments for not leading the antituberculosis campaign:

> In 1923 the death rate from tuberculosis for Colorado was 168 per 100,000, the highest of all [states in] the U.S. Registration Area. The death rate for Denver was 209 per 100,000, the second highest in the U.S. Registration Area. . . . A broad general view of the anti-tuberculosis campaign in Colorado reveals very clearly a sad delinquency on the part of the State and Municipal Health Departments, due most likely to insufficient funds. On the other hand, private organizations although almost overwhelmed, are carrying on a magnificent work everywhere.

The emphatic doctor denounced what he called the "sad muddle" of tuberculosis control and asserted the need for a municipal tuberculosis bureau. Many of the things Henry Sewall had proposed in 1907—including prompt reporting and registration of cases of tuberculosis, an anti-spitting ordinance, and regulations protecting the milk supply—were being neglected almost twenty years later. In 1925 the Denver Tuberculosis Association was calling for the enforcement of public health laws in the city. Although state and city laws existed, enforcement was lax.

Moreover, there was little in the way of provision of care for those without means. In a survey made for the Colorado Tuberculosis Association in 1928 it was established that few free beds in Denver existed: The TB ward at Denver General had eighty-two beds; Boulder County Hospital was the only other county hospital that had a ward for tuberculosis. There were seventy-five beds at Craig Colony and forty-three at Sands House. National hospitals with accommodations in Denver were the Jewish Consumptives' Relief Society, 300 beds; Ex-patients Home, 84; and the National Jewish Hospital, with 264 "open air rooms, classes, preventoria or day camps." Later, in a report to the Colorado Tuberculosis Association, Colorado was named as being "one of nine of the forty-eight states not making state provision for its own resident, indigent cases. The need of a state tuberculosis . . . sanatorium was clearly brought out. . . . One active case to every ninety-nine persons was discovered."

Throughout the country, hospitals and sanatoria were being built and open-air schools organized, but a state facility in Colorado remained an elusive goal. A model for treatment of the disease was Bellevue Hospital in New York City, where James Alexander Miller had persuaded the authorities that tuberculosis patients should be collected into a single division rather than scattered in different hospitals under supervision of Columbia, Cornell, and New York universities. This may have been the model Waring had in mind. However, a major difficulty in

Colorado was funding: The state could not be depended upon for either the initial cost or continued maintenance of such a facility. With this background, it is easier to understand what followed.

In 1903 Henry Porter had become ill in southern California and was taken to a hospital in Glendale run by the Seventh-day Adventists. He was impressed by the care he was given and surprised when a young therapist refused a gratuity. Twenty-five years later he entered a similar hospital in San Diego, the Paradise Valley Sanitarium, and again was impressed by the care. Although not a member of that church (he was a nominal Episcopalian himself), Porter invited the Seventh-day Adventists to run the hospital which he intended to open in Denver. In 1928 he looked at various sites and decided on one at what is now South Downing and East Harvard Avenue. He and his daughter, Dora Porter Mason, gave $315,000 and forty acres of land, thus establishing Porter Hospital. The cornerstone was laid in 1929, and the hospital opened on February 16, 1930. Later Porter and his daughter gave $50,000 for a nurses' residence.[20]

Three months after Porter Hospital opened, James Waring went to a meeting in Quebec and wrote to Ruth on May 14: "Tell Father Porter not to do anything about the sanatorium till I get there. There's so much to decide about that we must travel cautiously. It is very wonderful that he wants to do this for me." No record exists of conversations that took place between Ruth and her father, but the question is raised as to whether or not Waring hoped that his father-in-law might provide funds for a TB sanatorium. What is known is that Porter offered to build another hospital in addition to Porter Hospital; he was still a wealthy man. Anne Waring Maer remembers her parents "talking about Henry Porter wanting to build a hospital for my father. However, I believe my father remarked that running a hospital, as such, was not how he wished to spend his time and energy."

But there may have been more to the story. According to Dr. Stewart Taylor, professor emeritus of obstetrics and gynecology at the University of Colorado School of Medicine, Waring once said to him, "Stewart, do you know the biggest disappointment in my life? It was when my father-in-law built Porter Hospital instead of building something for the patients of Colorado General." There is no evidence that there was any breach in Waring's relationship with his father-in-law; he remained good friends with him, and they played billiards with Will Porter, Ruth's brother, almost weekly.

Not one to be dissuaded from a goal, in the years that followed Waring never gave up hope for a sanatorium. Ward A for tuberculosis patients at Colorado General Hospital opened in the 1930s; it was closed in 1941. Waring raised the question of reopening it for postgraduate education. When, in 1947, the state legislature turned down the request for a special tuberculosis facility in Colorado, Ward A for tuberculosis patients was reopened.

When Waring received the Florence Sabin Award in 1955, Mark Harrington, a leader in public health, said: "Dr. Waring lived through the period when the physicians fighting the cause of public health had to assume the leadership in their respective communities and take their places in the forefront of the struggle to obtain the facilities necessary. . . . Whether it was popular or unpopular, professionally expedient or inexpedient, likely to succeed or fail, make friends or provoke enmities, he was always willing to stand up and be counted for what he thought was right and would benefit the health of his fellow citizens."

Waring's social conscience and concern about the spread of disease seemed to echo his mother's concern for poor boys in her letters of long ago. In a crusade begun by Henry Sewall, Waring was looking for more facilities for victims of tuberculosis. He may have felt like Sisyphus rolling a stone uphill, but it was not for lack of trying that he never saw Colorado get the sanatorium he favored.

SMOKE COSTS CITY MILLIONS, SAYS DR., proclaims the headline in an undated Denver newspaper clipping. The article probably appeared about the mid-1920s, when Waring was president of the Denver Public Health Council. It told of his warning about smoke pollution as a menace to public health, estimating its cost to the city as $6,700,000 annually. In conclusion, Waring called for a citizens' smoke-abatement league.

The clipping illustrates Waring's concern with wider issues of public health. By the late 1920s, he had several forums in which to present his ideas. He was president of the Allied Health Council, probably in the mid-1920s; president of the Denver Public Health Council, 1925-1928; president of the Denver Sanatorium Association, 1926-1927; president of the Denver Medical Society, 1928-1929; and president of the Denver Tuberculosis Association, 1930. In 1928 he gained stature as a rising leader in his profession when he was inducted into the American College of Physicians. He co-founded the Colorado Society for Mental Hygiene with Franklin Ebaugh, a psychiatrist, and served as president, 1928-1929.

In a rousing speech to the Denver Medical Society on January 8, 1929—his presidential address—Waring spoke on public health reform. The society was fifty years old, he noted, with a roster of 570 members and "splendid library resources." And then he launched into his attack. The society, he said:

> threatens to evolve into nothing more than a forum for scientific discussion. . . . The average member discharges his obligations by . . . reading a paper occasionally and attending half a dozen meetings in which he usually doesn't take part. . . . In this age of preventive medicine and ever broadening social responsibilities . . . only a few members have taken an active interest individually in public-health affairs and until the past few years officially the society has held aloof and has done little or nothing in the advancement of all subjects connected with the healing art and public health.

Then he ripped into the low attendance at meetings in the past year, partly blaming a monotonous scientific program. He requested the medical school faculty's wholehearted interest in the conduct of the affairs of the society. He also called for varied programs of high scientific standards and more frequent presentation of patients in person. His sarcasm targeted the society's apathy: "Let some older and well informed members of this society review for you the rare occasions when this society has officially asserted itself in the interest of public health."

Waring then switched to a positive note and spoke of his hope that the joint dinner with the Denver Bar Association might become an annual affair. The event had been organized by Waring and his friend, Henry Wolcott Toll, president of the Denver Bar Association. Waring called for closer cooperation between the Denver Tuberculosis Society, the Colorado Tuberculosis Society, the Children's Hospital Outpatient Department, the Visiting Nurses Association, and other concerned groups.

A century before, Waring's great-grandfather, William Waring, had chastised the Georgia Medical Society for the poor health habits of the South. His grandfather, James Waring, also spoke out, alienating first the Georgia Medical Society and then many in Savannah with his rice farming directives. Now their descendant was speaking out, too. However, he believed that acting in concert with others would reap greater rewards than would the action of any one individual. Free from the bitterness of his earlier remarks, he closed his Denver Medical Society presidential address on a high note: "With generous spirit, high courage and with noble impulse, let us see to it that the county society fulfills its destiny as a progressive institution."

Although Waring's gravitation to the public health movement followed naturally enough from personal conviction, it is of note that Drs. Osler and Welch, the two professors who most influenced him at Johns Hopkins, also were actively involved in public health and in the antituberculosis movement in particular. Call it what one will—coincidence, synchronism, fate—James Waring seemed always to be near, in place and time, the men who were shaping the antituberculosis movement, and these men influenced his life.

Twenty-five years before Waring spoke out to the Denver Medical Society on public health, a tuberculosis exposition was convened in Baltimore under the auspices of the state Tuberculosis Committee with the State Board of Health Association. Prodded by William Osler, the governor of Maryland had taken the lead in championing the need for state involvement in fighting TB. The purpose of the exposition was to instruct the public about tuberculosis and necessary hygienic precautions to prevent its spread. Among those attending were Osler and Welch. Welch had helped to obtain a filtration plant for the city water supply and the delivery of pasteurized milk. Osler was concerned about the number of Johns Hopkins students who were not well and urged that their living conditions should be investigated, just as those of consumptive patients were investigated.

In the spring of 1905, when Waring was a freshman at Hopkins, the first meeting of the National Association for the Study and Prevention of Tuberculosis was held in nearby Washington, D.C. Edwin Trudeau of Saranac Lake was elected the first president, and Osler, one of the founders and a vice president, addressed the group. In 1907, two months after the diagnosis of Waring's illness, the third annual meeting of the National Association for the Study and Prevention of Tuberculosis was held, again in Washington. Among those attending were Trudeau, Gerald Webb of Colorado Springs, and Henry Sewall of Denver. Waring would have met Trudeau by then, but it would be a year or more before he met Webb and a few more before he met Sewall.

The antituberculosis movement might be said to have begun in New York City a decade before the turn of the century, led by Dr. Hermann Biggs, who called for legislation for sanitary reform. Dr. S. A. Knopf of that city was another leader in the movement. A rival group, led by Dr. Lawrence F. Flick of Philadelphia, began about the same time. This group had both lay and medical members, which helped to widen the rift between the two groups. A new organization, the National Tuberculosis Association (NTA), was established when Drs. Welch, Osler, Flick, and others bypassed both of the earlier competing groups and formed a truly national organization. They were pioneers in bringing together doctors and lay people to fight tuberculosis.

James Waring carried their cause forward. By the late 1920s, his reputation had spread beyond Colorado, and he was asked to speak to health workers in other cities. Dr. J. Arthur Myers wrote that in 1925 Waring went to Minneapolis to inspect a special school that had been developed for tuberculous children. "During this visit the Minneapolis workers were so impressed with Waring's wealth of knowledge, his scientific approach to the problem of tuberculosis . . . that thereafter, we looked upon him as a counselor. . . . Throughout the years, we frequently sought his advice on various problems." Myers cited Waring's "interest in protecting children against tuberculosis. . . . He was particularly desirous of seeing long-term studies conducted on children." In 1930 Waring helped instigate a parental and preschool health demonstration with the Parent-Teachers Association of the public schools. Eighty classes a month were held in twenty different schools to teach children and their parents good health habits.

By 1935, when elected president of the NTA, Waring had become a nationally recognized leader in the field. Through all the increasing responsibilities he was assuming at the medical school, tuberculosis—its cause and treatment—remained uppermost in his mind. Like his grandfather and great-grandfather, he never lost sight of the importance of work in public health.

7 | *Westerner*

PARENTS generally learn to nurture from their own parents. Discipline was strict in the new Waring family, for this is the way James Waring and Ruth Porter had been raised. Both daughters remember being made to sit "a long time"—perhaps as long as forty-five minutes—before an unfinished bowl of cereal or a plate of rejected vegetables, then having to go to bed if the food remained uneaten. Daughter Ruth remembers a choice of punishment: a spanking or bed. Occasionally, for a severe infraction, a hairbrush was used for a spanking, but not often. Writing to Ruth from a medical meeting in 1928, James urged, "Do not be too rigid. . . . I would not think of putting them to bed on orange juice! Plenty of patience—much encouragement, and firmness and consistency is all they need."

Waring's warmth as a father comes through in his letters. When he went to the Mayo Clinic in 1927 for an intestinal complaint, he wrote Anne: "Dear Teenykins, I send you my love and hope you are getting Big and Fat. Do give Mummie a goodnight kiss for me every night when you go to bed. Your loving Daddy." Anne later said of this time in her life: "He was loving and fun, with great whimsical humor, which we saw mainly at mealtime." She remembers her father as being tall, which is not quite the way Ruth remembers him, for she is tall herself. On a form he listed his height as being five feet, eleven inches. Anne, who inherited her father's brown eyes, more closely resembled her mother; Ruth grew to be taller than her mother.

A succession of nursemaids took care of the girls. One of the children's favorites was a jolly young woman named Verona, who entertained them by singing popular songs such as "Tiptoe through the Tulips," "Blue Skies," and "Barnacle Bill the Sailor." In September 1927 Ruth Waring went east to take Laurene to Smith College—girls did not travel unchaperoned in those days—and James was left at home, with a woman named Ireland caring for the children. He wrote his wife that the nursemaid was "a strict disciplinarian" and believed in iron-clad schedules. She was "a great talker—keeps up a running fire of conversation with the babies, [and] is learning also not to bully them too much over their meals. . . . [She] is quite energetic about taking them out to play with other children, which I think is an excellent plan." A few days later he wrote, "Miss Ireland sure does crack the whip, especially at mealtimes." Then about a month later, when Ruth was at home and he was in Kansas City, he wrote, "I do not approve of Miss Ireland's methods. I know you will be very gentle with her and agree with me to be guarded in our criticism of her after she has gone. . . . Do not be too rigid with that thirty-minute stuff [probably referring to keeping them at the table until they ate their food] with the Babies. Stretch the time somewhat—if necessary."

The family was seldom without a couple of little dogs, among them a much-loved mongrel, Teddy; a Scottie named Mackie; and two generations of Welsh terriers called Roger and Rowdy. Still, it was not a house for childish antics. Anne harbored regrets that she was not allowed to slide down the banisters because of possible damage to tapestries that hung on them. The girls were expected to be quiet for their father, which explains why they were not encouraged to bring playmates home from school and why they grew up feeling a bit lonely. The sisters spent hours reading in the playroom, romping on the jungle gym in the garden, or playing on the third floor of their home with marionettes and puppets made at school. With memories of not being allowed to make a mess, Anne remarked that when her own sons were small, she encouraged them to create with clay and to paint, with no concern for the spills that go with such activity.

In 1928 Waring's mother developed an abdominal problem and was operated on by Dr. George Packard. Although she was seventy years old, she came through the operation but was now quite frail. The experience, she wrote Antonio, had strengthened her faith. Pondering the death of Edith Cavell, the English World War I nurse who had been executed by the Germans for trying to rescue English prisoners, she wrote: "Standing as I do in view of God and Eternity, I realize that Patriotism is not enough. I must have no hatred nor bitterness toward anyone. . . . It was a flash of light to me—love for my children was not enough—when I pass through 'the valley' I must appear to the other side with only forgiveness and love on my face and in my heart truly truly, not just indifference—and this is my task for the days that are left." In another letter, she wrote of destroying old letters in the attic of the Savannah house. She and Minna returned to Savannah each winter. "Sad, old letters have torn my heart today and even made the sunlight dark."

In April 1929 Waring returned to Savannah for his first visit in years. The family and friends looked old, he wrote Ruth, "especially the gals." Little Anne's birthday was on April 7, and he wrote Ruth to tell his daughter of the happiness she had brought them. In Savannah he became the child again in memory, walking by the old Waring house at 3 Perry Street. "It was strange to stand on the pavement outside the old house and gaze through the iron fence at the garden where I played as a child," he wrote. "So much has changed, and that change so radical, that the old places seem hardly the same." Looking at the house with all its memories, he may have turned his thoughts to his father, about whom he knew so little. An official notice had reached the two Waring brothers from Spain—the precise year is not known—advising them that Antonio Gogorza had died and had bequeathed some land to them. They had written back to say they would not accept their father's bequest.[21]

James Waring's father was always a taboo subject within the family in Denver—at least any discussion of him with his daughters—just as it had been in Savannah. Yet he may have felt some ambivalence in his secrecy. His biography in James H. Baker's and LeRoy R. Hafen's *History of Colorado* (1927) begins: "Dr. James Johnston Waring, a physician of notable scientific attainments, is practicing in Denver and has become widely known through his contributions to medical literature. He was born August 11, 1883, in Savannah, Georgia, and is a son of Antonio de Gogorza, a native of Spain, and Annie Johnston Waring, who was also born in the city of Savannah."

Similarly, Waring had named his father on the form sent out in 1914 by the decentennial committee of the Yale-Sheffield class of 1904. However, when he sent in the form for his Yale class's twenty-fifth reunion in 1929, there was no mention of his father. In listing his work, his family, and his interests, he did not mention in his reply—after all, it was just a college alumni form—the tremendous amount of work he was able to accomplish despite having always to measure his limited energy so carefully. He did not say that at last he was in control of his life and his career, speaking out increasingly and forcefully on subjects that mattered to him. Nor did he tell his former classmates that he had a wife whom he loved and who loved him without reservation, accepting his fragile health and dedicating herself to taking care of him, and that he had two bright, healthy little girls. From his letters it is apparent he was happier than he had ever been before, but how could he tell that to the class of 1904?

A facade of pleasantness existed between the Porters and Waring's mother and Aunt Minna, but relations were strained between them. In a 1924 letter, Annie wrote Antonio: "Minna, Alston and I, Jim and Ruth, dined with the Will Porters. Minna went for Jim's sake. She did not want to go, but Jim said he did like his family 'to appear' sometimes, to support him. Mr. and Mrs. Porter made a real effort and we met them half way." A misalignment between the more direct ways of the West and the polite customs of the South may have been at fault, or it may have been simply a difference in temperaments.

Envy was not a part of Annie's or Minna's makeup; on the contrary, Annie's letters to Antonio showed that material things meant increasingly less and less to her. She wanted the two families to get along together. "Life is too short to add to its difficulty and I am more and more impressed with its continuity and it would fill me with shame to carry over any enmity, even the more trivial," she wrote Antonio. "I want you to know this now. I must have only love and light on my face when I cross over from this land to that." As for Minna, while wintering in Savannah in 1925 she wrote Jim: "I understand and know how to talk to people in the South and can't talk to Western people. Southern people love talking and they respond to anyone. At this boarding house one is introduced to anyone standing by and all talk. That is the South. And that is why we mind loneliness."

Houstoun Waring remembers Aunt Minna as being a hilarious storyteller: "She could retell a story and all would be on the floor laughing." On a trip to England in 1926, Minna and Annie took the adventurous step of flying across the English Channel to France because all the bookings on the channel steamer were taken because of the imminent general strike. It was a turbulent crossing, both were sick, and they had a forced landing. The fact that they would even consider taking such a wild flight shows the difference between them and the Porters, whose lives were governed by a carefully regimented, predictable routine. "You could set your watch and calendars by the Porters," says a great-granddaughter. "They were the most disciplined people who ever existed." In contrast to Minna, Ruth's mother, Laura Smith Porter, would have had stories to tell of her parents' trek west in a covered wagon and of the privations that accompanied such a venture. Such memories tended to produce stoics, people who kept a tight rein on their emotions.

Henry and Laura Porter were eighty-one and seventy, respectively, when James Waring married their daughter, and thus a pronounced generation gap existed when Ruth and Anne were old enough to get to know their grandparents. Anne recalls Sundays at the Porters'—915 Vine Street, near the Warings'—as being interminable; few games were allowed. "Children should be seen and not heard" was the rule. Grandfather Porter wanted a ballroom at 915 Vine but compromised and settled for a billiard room. Sometimes Grandmother Porter took the children out to ride with her, and in the back seat of the Packard, with the chauffeur at the wheel, they drove through suburban Denver. Passing through Cheesman Park, the little girls could never stop and join other children playing there. They had few playmates and wished they had more.

Loneliness occasionally bothered the girls' father, too, especially when his wife was away and he was at home. At these times he opened up his heart to Ruth: "I get more dependent upon your love and loyal support every day." In February 1927 when Ruth and the children were in Pasadena, he wrote that the house was "lifeless" and that he was uneasy about her and the little ones because he had heard of heavy rains in California: "Sunday and everything quiet! Business poor! . . . Sitting in the sun-room at [the] victrola playing 'Caprice Viennois'! I miss you excruciatingly. . . . I was terribly disappointed not to hear yesterday. Do send me some word every day!" On another occasion when Ruth was away but the children—then very small—were at home, he wrote, "My wings are too thin and scrawny for little chick-a-biddies to shelter under."

Waring felt great pride that neither of his daughters ever tested positive for tuberculosis. However, both girls suffered the usual childhood illnesses. In 1928 Ruth went to Bermuda with some friends, leaving James with the children and a nursemaid. As luck would have it, the "Babies" (he always capitalized the word) were sick in bed, with fevers, for three days. Then, after displaying normal temperatures, they were sick again and coughing. He called in another doctor. The sitter caught the bug, too, and had to leave, but Grandmother Waring came regularly to supervise.

Ruth Waring Halpenny recalls these illnesses as having been "miserable." The first was measles, and she recalls not being able to tolerate any light; the second was whooping cough. After about a week, both girls were well again, but their father was exhausted from anxiety. He wrote Ruth, "Anne much better, chipper as a lark. . . . Ruth eating splendidly. Am feeling better myself but always anxious about you and my Babies when you are away. Have a good time—you deserved the vacation and I do not begrudge it—but it's lonely when you are away."

Such words of devotion and dependence were important to Ruth, according to Polly Riedeburg Plesset, who lived across the street from the Warings from age three until she went away to college. Ruth and Anne, two and three years younger than she, were her earliest friends.

"She needed him," she says of Ruth. "She put up a brave front; only he saw that vulnerable side. They were both very much in love."

"IF GRALAND [Country Day] School is a success I don't know but what we ought to send them there this winter," James wrote Ruth in 1927, "more for the social contacts than anything else." The little girls were, in fact, only four and three when the new Country Day school opened with twenty-three boys and twenty-eight girls. Ruth and Anne were not yet of school age when their mother and Abby Staunton (Mrs. Morrison) Shafroth helped found the school. Virginia Shafroth Newton, a daughter of the Shafroths, recalls that there was first a kindergarten on Franklin Street near East Eighth Avenue in Denver in about 1925. Ruth Waring and Abby Staunton Shafroth talked to the two women who ran the school, Grace Laird and Virginia Braswell; then they wrote and visited the Shady Hill School in Cambridge, Massachusetts, where they persuaded Georgia Nelson to come to Denver to help start Graland, operating out of a small house at 1012 Pennsylvania until a school could be built. Virginia Newton states that James Waring and Morrison Shafroth "were somewhat skeptical that their wives could start a school but changed their minds when they returned from a visit to *The Denver Post* with a $10,000 check," Among others who helped in the fundraising were Mrs. Leroy McWhinney, Mrs. Henry Toll, and Mrs. Fred Lanagan.

Ruth (Mrs. Paul) Gorham has been associated with the school since 1930, mainly as a teacher, and today serves with the school's development staff, maintaining relationships with alumni. She has provided a history of the school that tells how Grace Laird and Virginia Braswell started with a preschool on Colfax Avenue between Cook and Madison streets in 1924 before the move in 1925 to "the Green House" at 773 Franklin Street, providing the first grade of the new school. She recalls that James Waring wanted the school located east and south of the city, on high ground, with plenty of sunshine. Before the land was acquired in 1927, the founders wrote: "The ideal location would be a ten-acre tract situated southeast of the city limits. This would be high land sloping to the southwest, thus assuring a maximum of sunlight and affording an unobstructed view of the mountain ranges, and being easily accessible from the city. Here, also, the air is free from smoke and dust." James Waring's belief in the benefits of sunshine was shared by the administration of Graland Country Day School: For many years, after lunch and in good weather, the children rested on portable cots on the spacious flat roof adjacent to the gymnasium.

Ruth Gorham and Dr. Henry Toll, Jr., recall hearing that the Warings walked over to see Mrs. Verner Z. Reed, who lived nearby, and returned with the deed (or at least assurance of it) to the land on which the school eventually was located. Ruth Porter Waring was among the fifteen persons who formed the corporation named on the certificate issued by the state, dated July 23, 1927. When ground was broken at First and Birch streets in 1927, daughter Anne, age three, dug the first shovelful of dirt. All the land around the school was prairie; Clermont Street and East Ellsworth Avenue comprise the other sides of the block. Jacques Benedict, again, was the architect. Virginia Newton gives an idea of how undeveloped the area was in the 1930s: Once a week she and her sister Ellen rode horses to school from their farm, north of what is now Belleview Avenue and east of University. After school they would ride back home with the Hottentot Riding Club. When they studied knighthood—a Graland tradition—they used their horses as part of the pageantry.

Anne tells of what Graland instilled: intellectual curiosity, freedom of expression, independence, love of books. Cooperation rather than competition was emphasized. Another happy memory is of Georgia Nelson, headmistress, who read to the children after lunch and also taught when there was a need. Georgia Nelson was an inspiration to all. Not only had Ruth Waring and Abby Staunton Shafroth chosen the right person to run the school but, with other parents, they also had been successful in fundraising to start the school.

With both parents maintaining such full schedules, extra help was needed around the house. A man, Erickson, was hired by the Warings to be gardener and do errands. One of Ruth's and Anne's great embarrassments as children was being driven to school by Erickson on those occasions when their mother was busy at meetings and unavailable to drive them. Not wanting to have their classmates see them being chauffeured, they would duck down below the windows.

The family took weekend excursions to Hilltop, the mountain house on Upper Bear Creek in Evergreen. They avoided going in July and August, when James and Ruth found their susceptibility to hay fever at its height. Hilltop, an hour's drive from Denver, stood on a slope covered with pine and aspen and had a view of the Front Range. There was a screened-in porch in a separate building especially for Waring. An arched doorway led into a porch, which opened into a big living room. Both the main floor and the upstairs contained two bedrooms. The dining room, with its bay windows, had a glorious view of the mountains to the west. The pine trees on the hills were good for the games of childhood, as were two wonderful large rock formations that became castles, ships, hotels.

Mary Barkalow Joyce, whose family was lent the use of Hilltop on several occasions when she was a child, recalls staying at

> this heavenly summer place in the month of July for three summers, 1924 to 1926. . . . [We played] wonderful games of Run-Sheep-Run and Kick the Can with our neighbors as well as games in the house, Charades and lots of reading out loud by the stone fireplace in the evenings. We children learned to lure the two horses, Goldy and Buck, from the pasture into the barn, where we learned to saddle and bridle them and then take off on mountain trails. . . . The view from Hilltop was spectacular. We looked out on what was then known as the Bendemere Valley: rolling green meadows interrupted by the meanderings of the blue, laced with white, Bear Creek, as it tumbled over rocky surfaces. Mount Evans was the focal point of that view and a very cherished visual sight in my memory today. As a little girl I often tried to capture that view in a drawing or painting.

When Anne thinks of her father fishing, she envisions him in his favorite Stetson hat with a braided horsehair hatband. Anne and Ruth diligently unraveled horsehairs from rough wooden fences against which the horses had rubbed or occasionally took them directly from an animal's tail when a special color was needed. The hat still exists. Encircling the crown is a series of vignettes, painted in oil colors by western artist Joe D. Young, of cows, calves, bucking broncos, and cowboys. James Waring's fishing attire—including a Navajo bolo, an old Zuni ring, and a red bandanna for drying flies as well as his hands—showed his love for the West.

Favorite fishing retreats were in Wyoming: Eaton's Ranch near Sheridan and the Bar A Ranch near Encampment. Every summer in the 1930s and 1940s he tried to spend a couple of weeks at a ranch with his family. One of daughter Ruth's early memories is of making a wooden waterwheel on a stream with her father and Anne. On these vacations, his fragile health was momentarily pushed aside, and both daughters recall his humor, lightheartedness, and teasing. Antonio, who shared his brother's passion for fishing, frequently joined them for these outings, sometimes accompanied by other members of his family: his wife Sue, sons Antonio Jr. and Will, and daughter Anne. The Waring girls had riotous times when Uncle Antonio and their cousins arrived, says Anne Waring Maer, who recalls the many summers she helped her uncle grease his fishing line after first carefully winding it around the big Russian olive trees in their garden.

Since the family wanted a quiet retreat in the country closer than Hilltop, in the late 1920s they had Jacques Benedict build a more accessible country house for them in Arapahoe County, south of Denver, in what is now Greenwood Village. "Contract signed and house started. Aren't you thrilled?" Waring wrote Ruth in October 1928.

The house Benedict designed was perfect for the site, with a sweeping view of the mountains to the west. They named it Green Meadows. Its classic lines fit in well with the rolling countryside of alfalfa fields. Today, magnificent trees surround the house; nearby is a lateral of the old High Line Canal, built decades earlier to irrigate the orchards and farmlands surrounding Denver. Anne remembers meadowlarks singing their lovely song. Many birds are attracted to the area, including magpies, kestrels, Canada geese, red-tailed hawks, seagulls, and mallard ducks. Waring raised chickens, guinea hens, and other fowl with the help of a tenant farmer, Joe Lind, just as years before he had raised chickens in Colorado Springs. Two horses were kept for the children, who loved riding along the canal.

The Farm, as they referred to the property—originally sixty acres—became James's domain, just as 910 Gaylord was Ruth's. He had a chaise lounge similar to the ones he had in town and at Hilltop, on which he would rest on a porch after lunch, regardless of weather. Besides his usual fare of medical journals, medical history, and other more weighty reading, he liked to relax with the *Saturday Evening Post.*

At The Farm, their closest neighbors were Allen and Emma True. The Trues bought land together with the Warings, and Allen True had a house and studio built on the property. After the Trues were divorced and the land divided, the studio ended up with the Warings and served double-duty as a place for parties, just the right size for square dances. Waring took special pleasure in the player piano, and charades was a favorite game. At one time Ruth had a badminton court inside, and later a tennis court was added outdoors for Ruth and Anne.

Each Fourth of July, the family held a spectacular party at The Farm. Ruth, a marvelous hostess, would be in her element: Normally reserved, she showed a different side for this annual affair. Friends such as Henry and Cyrena Toll came with their families, and their son, Henry Toll Jr., recalls the fun he had as a child at the Warings' parties. Imagine the setting: a soft breeze coming over the fields, the towering cottonwoods swaying on the High Line Canal to the southeast, with a brilliant sunset over Mount Evans to the west; mallards flying overhead to a nearby pond, barnyard sounds competing with the laughter of the guests; Waring in a chef's hat, cooking hamburgers on the grill; then—best of all—fireworks after sundown!

But the party for which the Warings became best known was their annual Christmas Eve party at 910 Gaylord Street. Until Ruth and Anne were in their mid-teens, the party was only for adults. As young girls, Anne and Ruth would peek down through the stair railing to see the seventy-five or so people gathered below. At dinnertime, the tradition was for Henry Toll Sr., Morrison Shafroth, and James Waring to don chefs' caps and ceremoniously carry in the platters—Toll would carry the turkey, Waring the ham, and Shafroth the pig. Ruth's eggnog and cake, shaped like a lamb, followed dinner, and more guests would arrive to sing carols. Later, when the red songbooks were distributed, the familiar favorites would help put the two little girls to sleep upstairs. Their mother accompanied the carolers on one of the grand pianos, while another guest, usually Erma Brodhead, played the other. A tall tree reached to the ceiling, with lights reflecting off many-colored foil, and some ornaments belonging to Ruth's mother and grandmother. On these occasions the details of Allen True's painted ceiling, the handsome fireplace designed by Jacques Benedict, all the other carefully planned features, and the big room itself—normally too formal and too large for a small family—seemed just right.

Flowers were an integral part of Ruth Porter Waring's life. She was serious enough about gardening to join the Garden Club of Denver in 1917. After she married she grew flowers with the aid of a gardener, adding a greenhouse to 910 Gaylord Street near the property line of what today is the Denver Botanic Gardens. James did his pollen studies in the greenhouse early in their marriage; through the years he was in the habit of wearing a flower in his buttonhole, often a red carnation, from Ruth's greenhouse. In time she turned to cultivating orchids.

Ruth ran the household for the health and well-being of her husband, providing the quiet and rest he needed to conserve his strength. She was the consummate hostess, yet she was the quiet one, he the gregarious one. She planned the meals, paid the bills, oversaw the staff, and worked hard in her garden. Her forte was volunteer work. "Glad you are out of the Red Cross and hope the bookkeeping will soon be finished," her sister Dora (Dodie) Mason wrote her in March 1933. Ruth was devoted to Dodie.

In a review of a biography of William Osler in "Library Notes," Waring wrote: "Mrs. Osler radiated an efficiency that made any man coming under her dominion feel that he was carefree in all mundane matters. There is not the least doubt that he was an extraordinarily well watched over and well looked after saint." He might have been writing about his own Ruth and the care with which she looked after him.

Ruth's dedication to making her husband's life run smoothly made her daughters feel somewhat left out. Because their father needed quiet time in the house, the girls were not encouraged to bring friends home from school. Anne recalls her mother's sharpness if she interrupted her at her desk. In contrast, she says her father would put down what he was doing if she came to him to talk or ask a question. Her father always looked things up when the family had dinner; reference books were shelved just outside the dining room. "He taught me the value of doing this and so I continued the habit with my two sons," she says.

Despite the growing pains and the frustrations of childhood, Ruth and Anne adored their parents. Anne was overtaken by homesickness when she and Ruth went away to camp in summer. In June 1933, when she was nine, she wrote to her father: "You don't know how much I miss you. And how much I love you dear daddy." To her mother, June 1934: "Dear Mother, I don't want to stay here. . . . I do so long for home. Please right [*sic*] me in printing. Love, Anne." Although Ruth did not seem to mind the camp, the following summer Anne told her mother, "I am getting very homesick and miss you a lot. I do not like it well here [worst of all was having to clean the outdoor latrines]. . . . I hope I can come home."

Although James Waring was gaining a wider coterie of medical friends from coast to coast by attending meetings, he and Ruth had an assortment of nonmedical friends in Denver. The Arthur Sayre Brodheads and the Warings often did things together. Anne recalls the time that the Brodheads and her parents, attending the theater together, sat behind a woman who was wearing a low-cut dress, showing off the creamy white skin of her back to advantage. Her father turned to Sayre Brodhead and said, "'Do you prefer the white meat of chicken?'" (Perhaps the lady in the low cut dress provided the inspiration for Ruth when, at a costume party on a Great Lakes tour boat with her family, she wore a evening dress with a low-cut back. James painted a "face" on her back, and when she moved her shoulders, she produced amusing expressions.) Henry and Cyrena Toll and Morrison and Abby Staunton Shafroth were also among the Warings' close friends, as were Charles and Eleanor Emery, Leroy and Alice McWhinney, Henry and Olga Riedeburg, and the Daniel Milletts.

Waring belonged to the Cactus Club, an all-male, and for the most

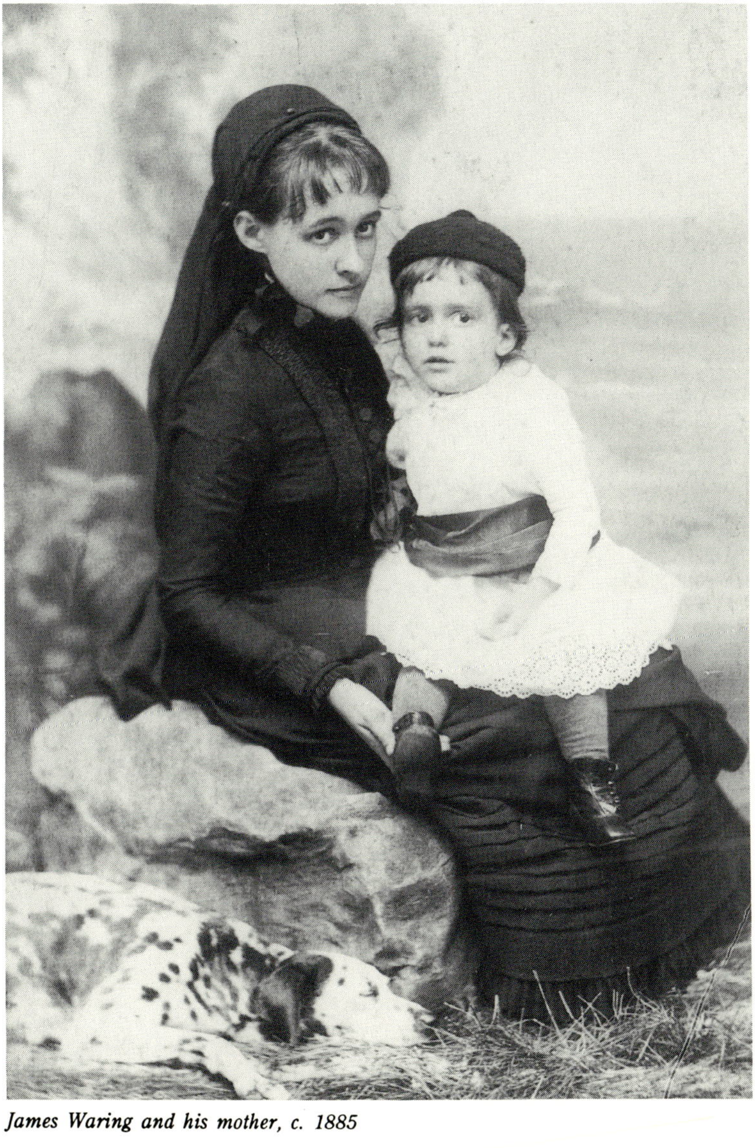

James Waring and his mother, c. 1885

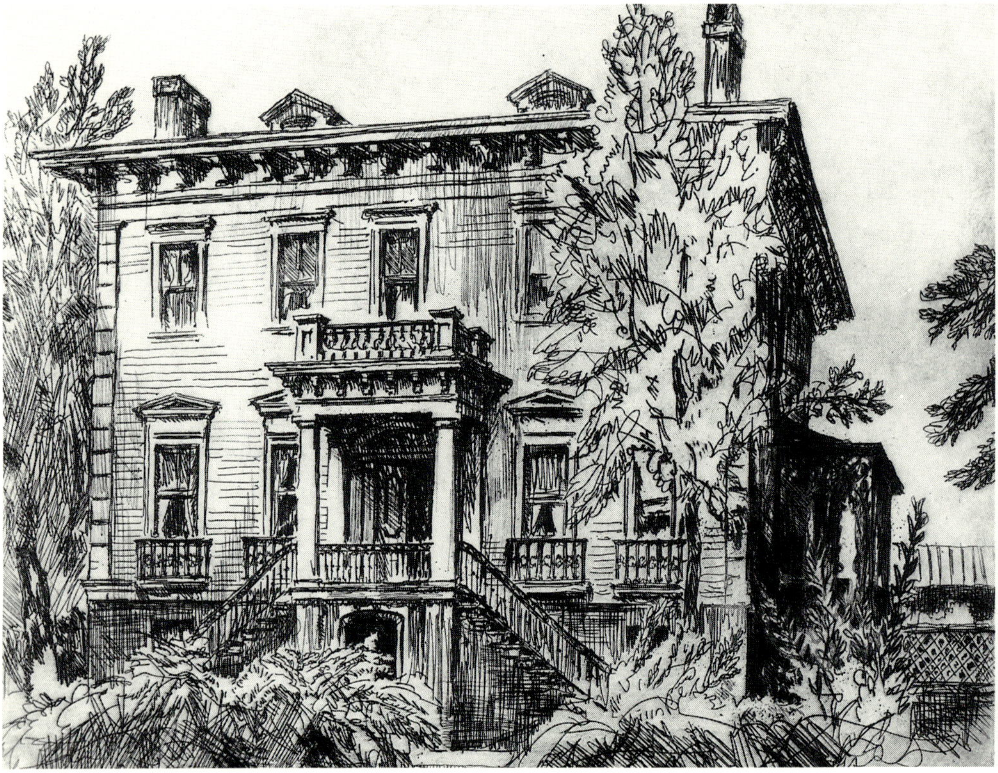

3 Perry Street, Savannah, Georgia, the home of Waring's maternal grandfather, James J. Waring, M.D.

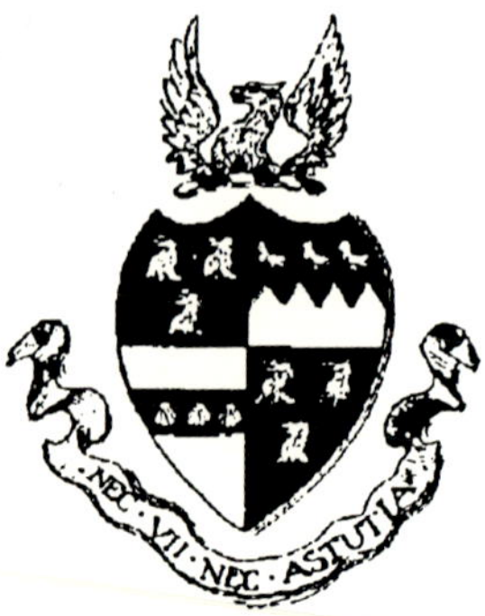

Waring coat of arms

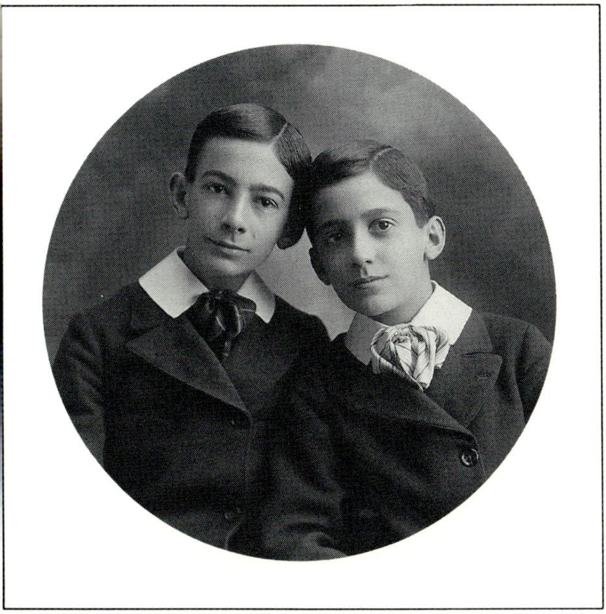

Brothers Antonio ("Tono") and James ("Jimmy")

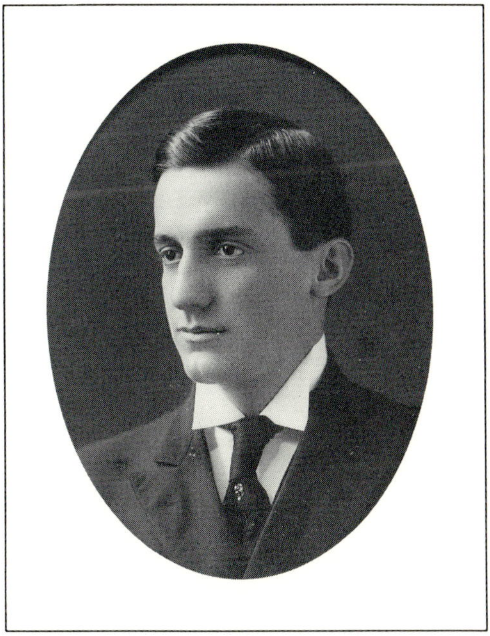

Jim Waring at Yale Sheffield Scientific School

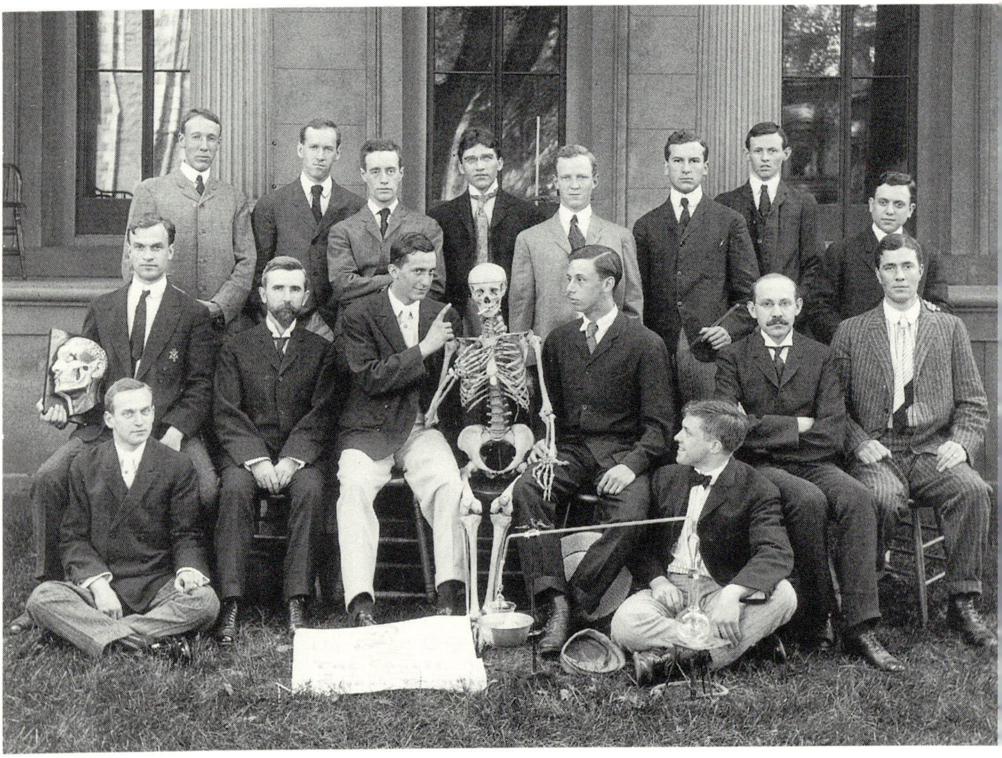

Jim Waring (seated, pointing at skeleton) and fellow graduates of the pre-med course at Yale Sheffield Scientific School, 1904. The sign reads: "The course that made Sheff famous."

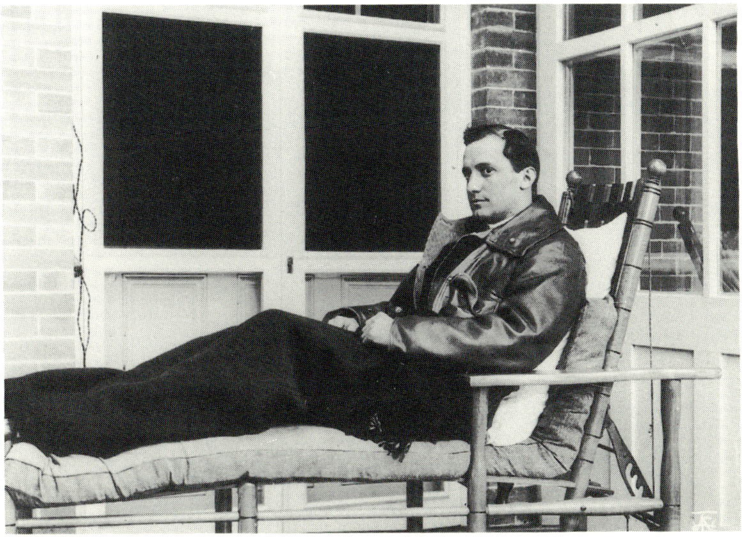

At the Trudeau Sanitarium, Saranac Lake, New York, 1907

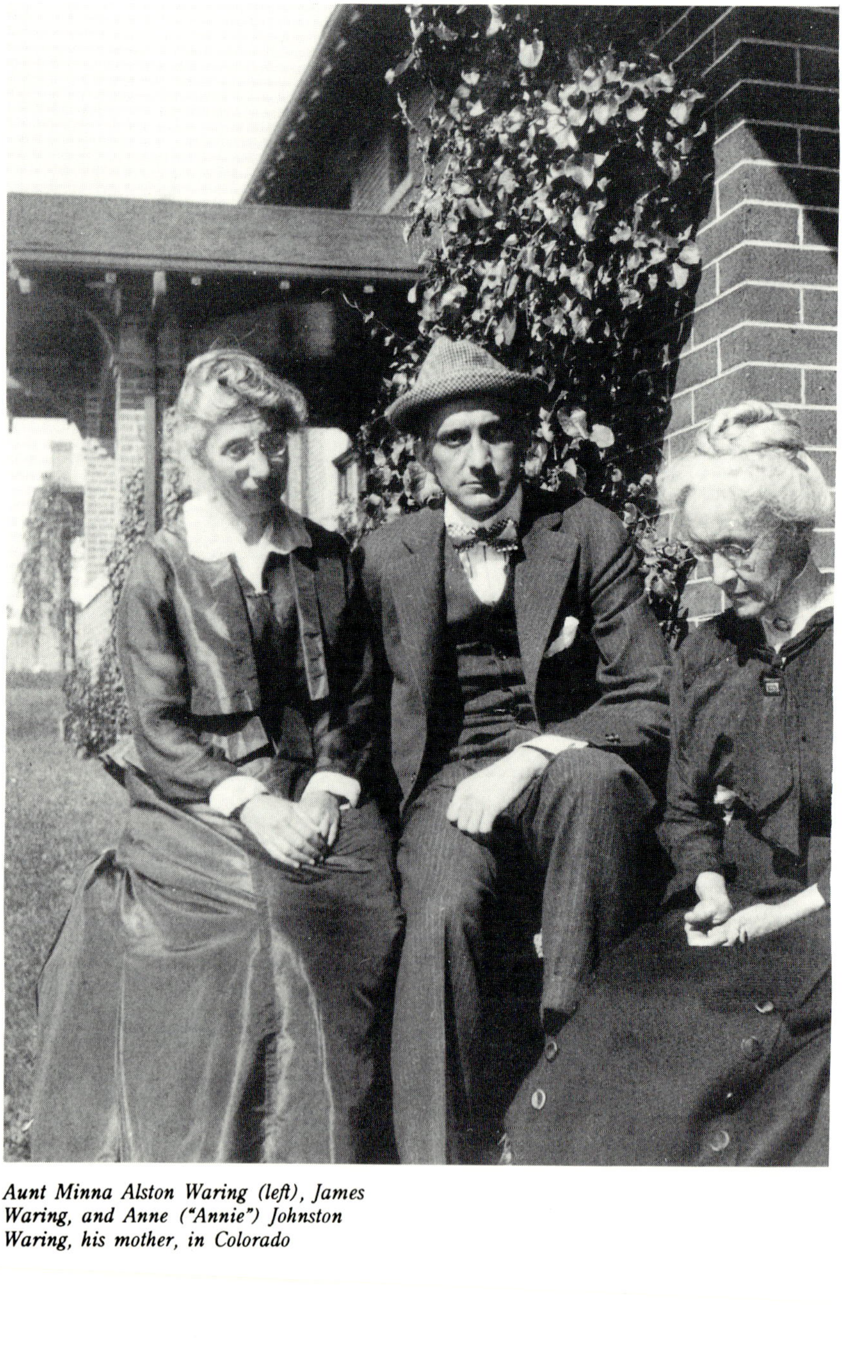

Aunt Minna Alston Waring (left), James Waring, and Anne ("Annie") Johnston Waring, his mother, in Colorado

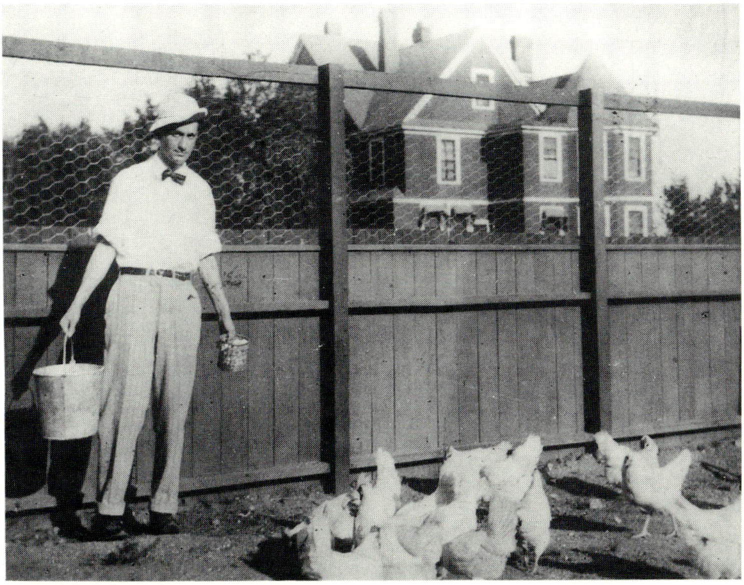

Waring and his hobby, Colorado Springs, c. 1910

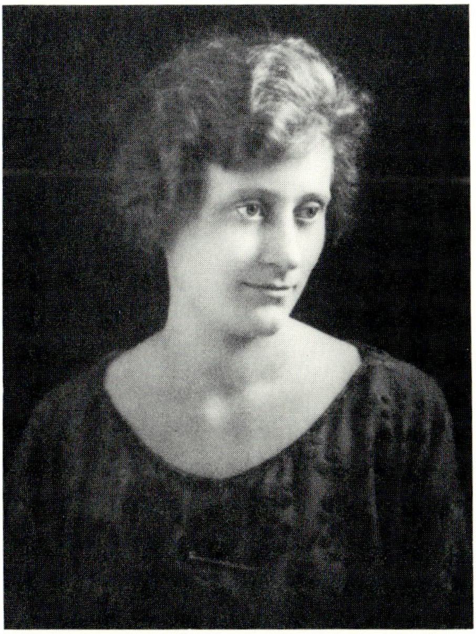

Waring's fiancée, Ruth Porter, c. 1921

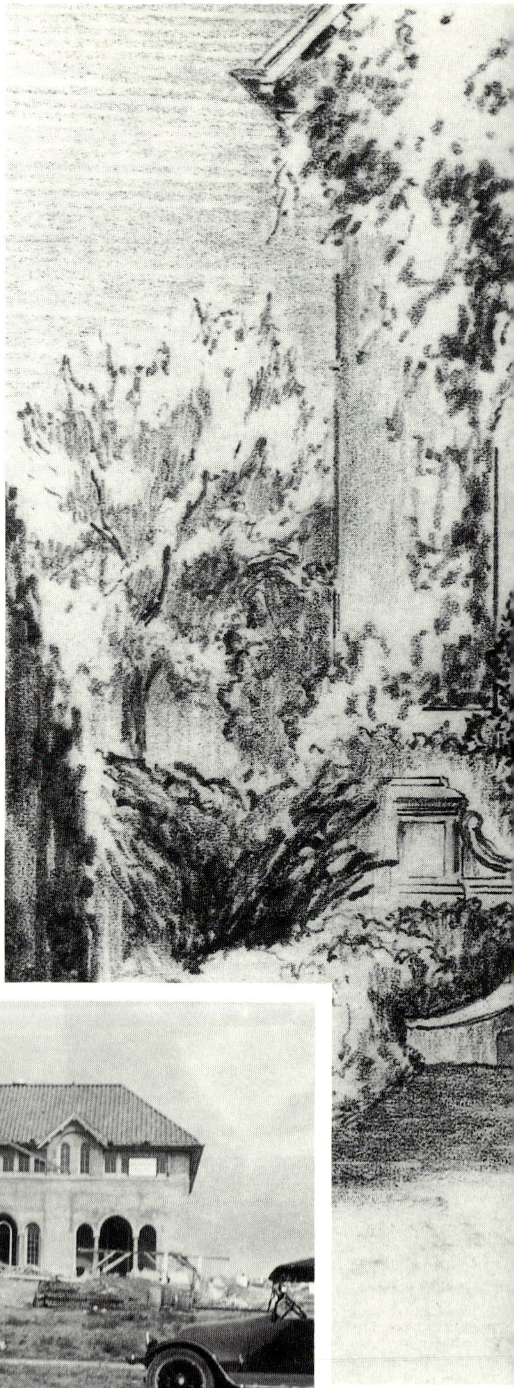

Architect Jules Jacques Benedict's detailed sketch of 910 Gaylord Street, Denver, and (inset) the house under construction, c. 1922

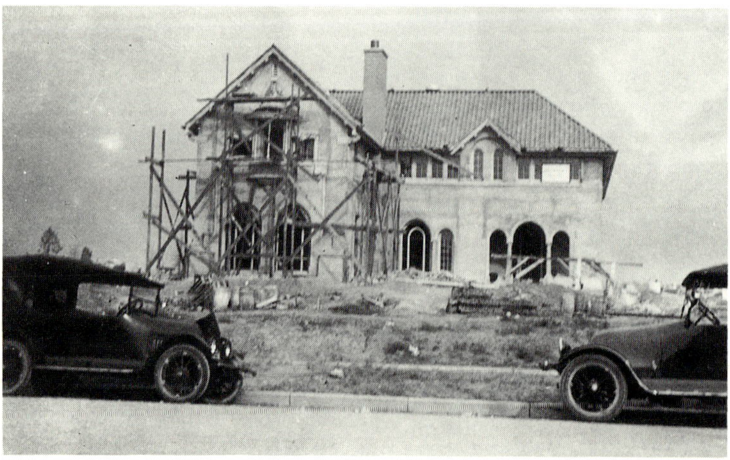

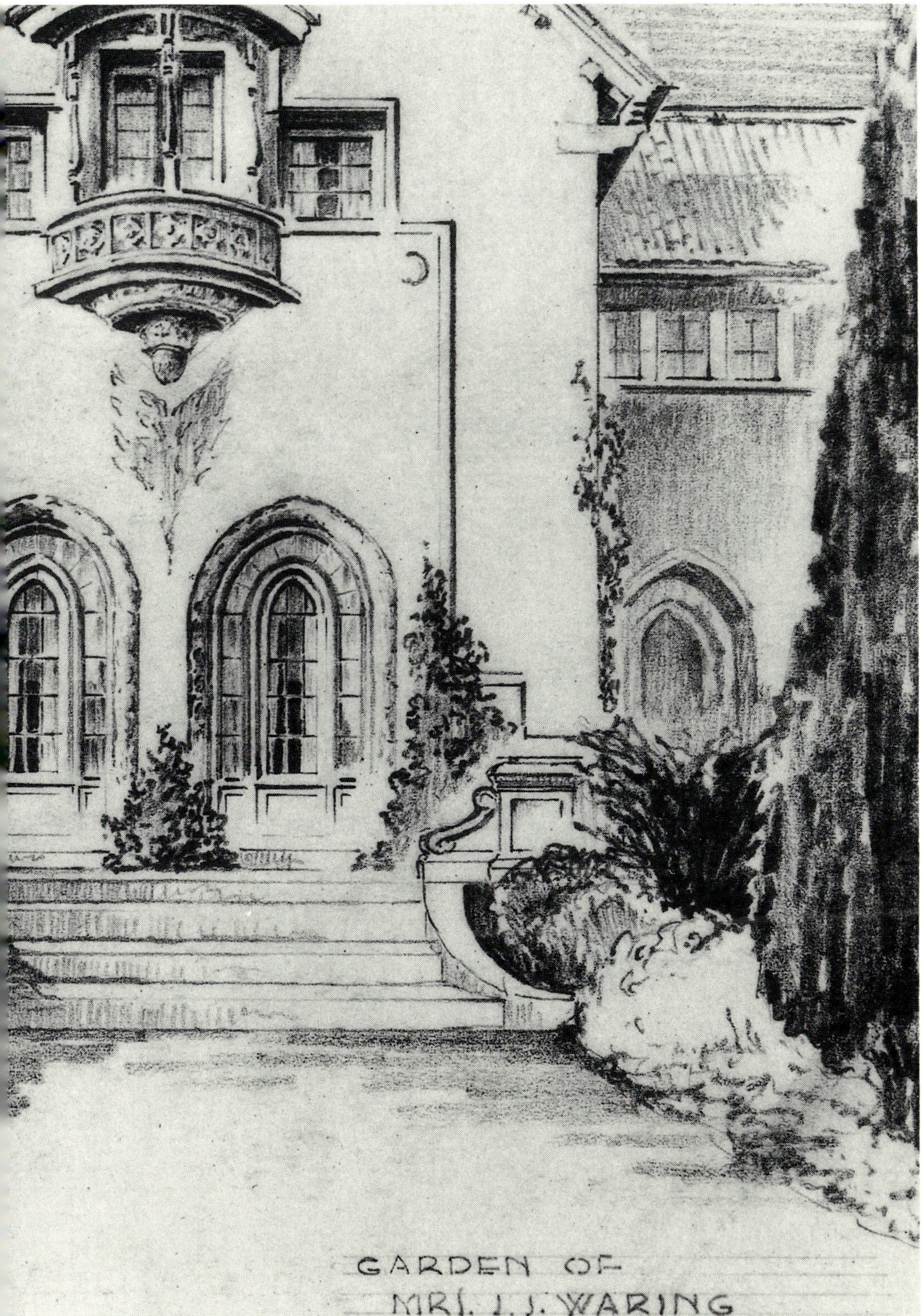
GARDEN OF
MRS. J. J. WARING

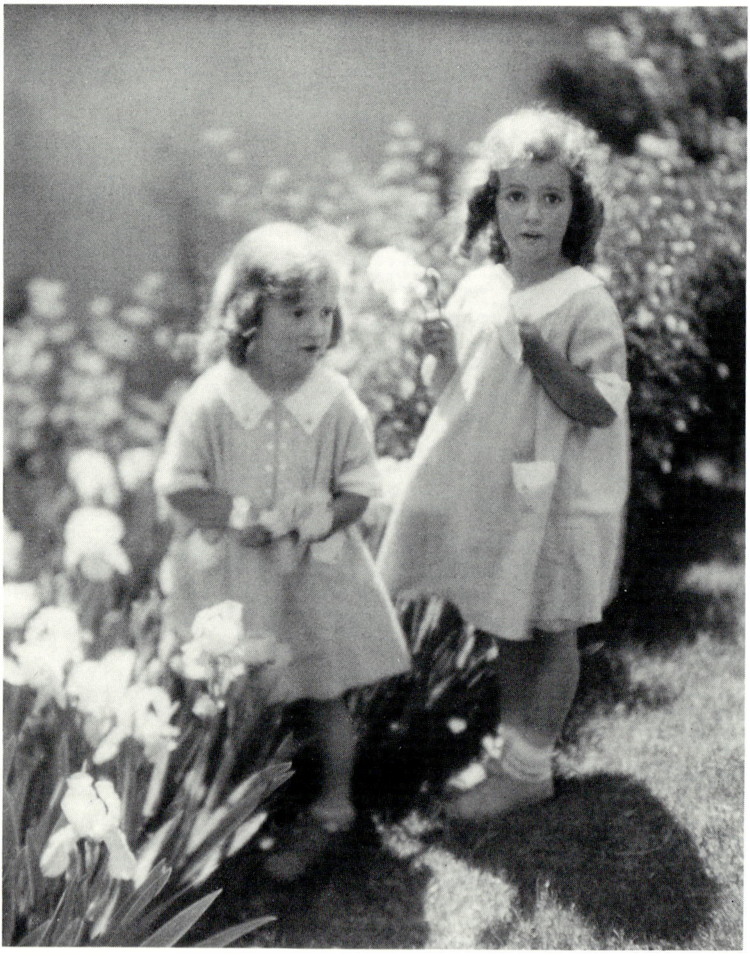

Laura Gilpin photograph of (left) Anne ("Teeny") and Ruth ("Bebe") Waring at 910 Gaylord Street

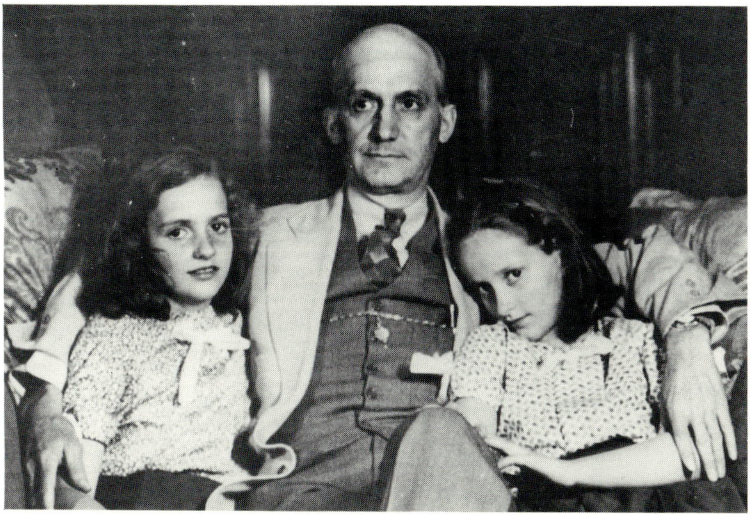

James Waring with daughters
Ruth (left) and Anne

Etching of cowboy by Joe D. Young,
a favorite artist of Waring's

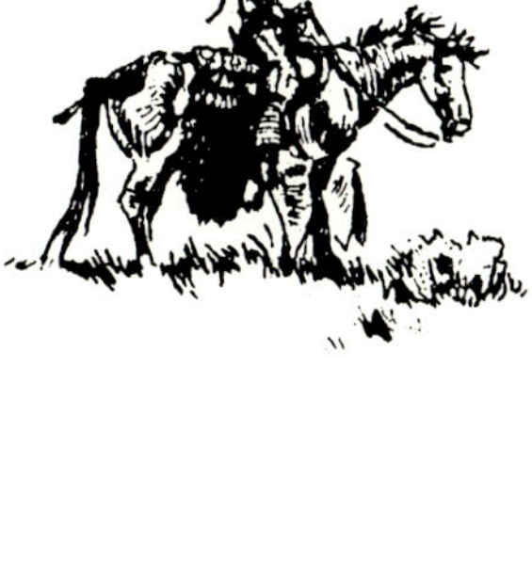

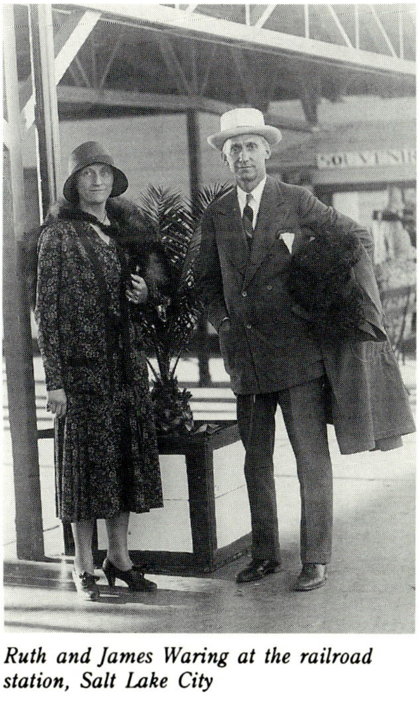

Ruth and James Waring at the railroad
station, Salt Lake City

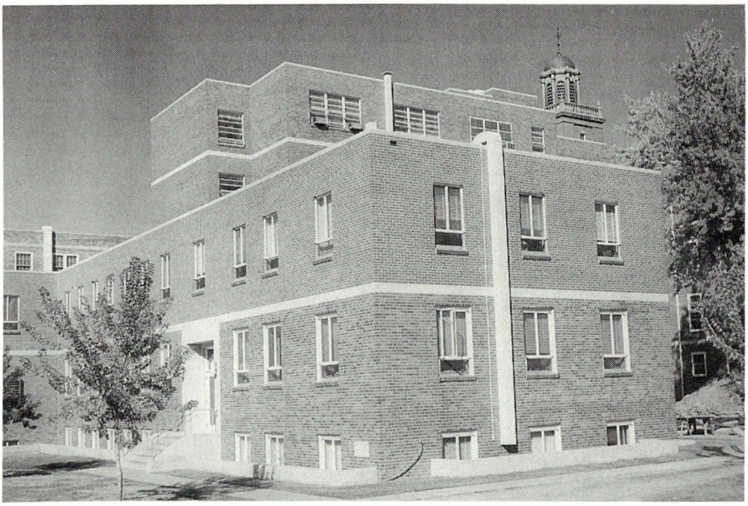

The Gerald B. Webb Memorial Building, early 1960s, before fourth and fifth floors were added. After several name changes, the institute is today the Webb-Waring Institute for Biomedical Research.

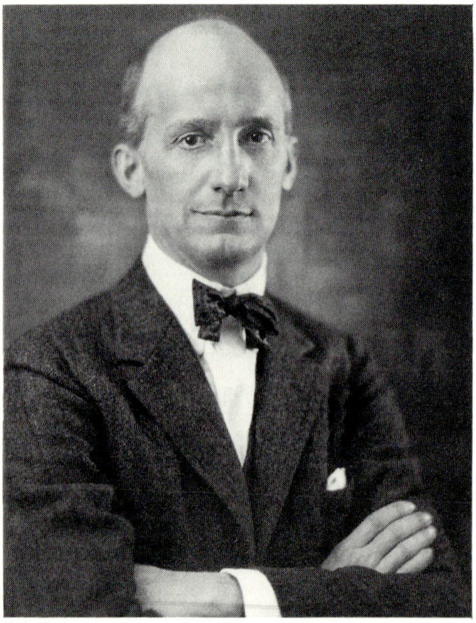

Waring at about the time he became chairman of the Department of Medicine, University of Colorado School of Medicine

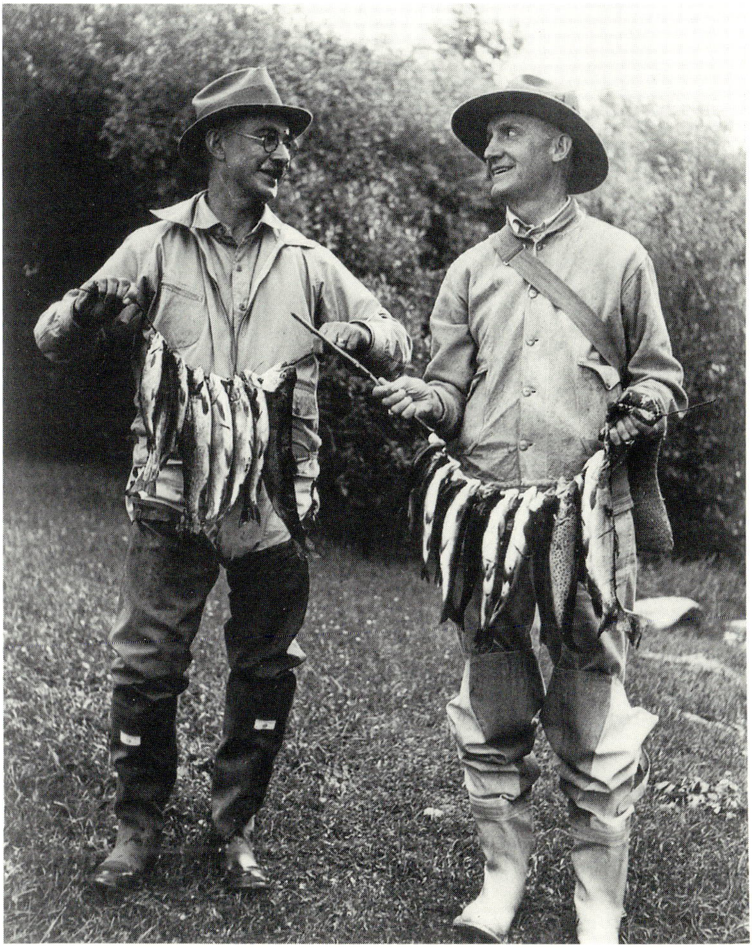

Brothers Tono and Jim

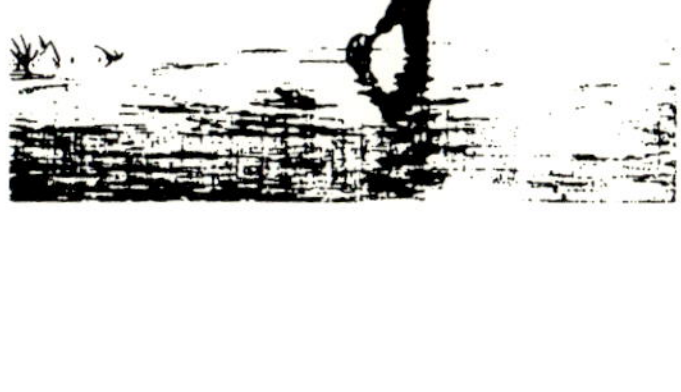

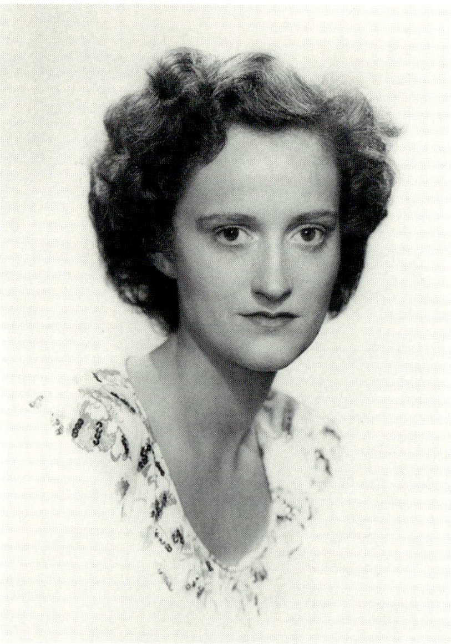

Anne Waring

Ruth Waring

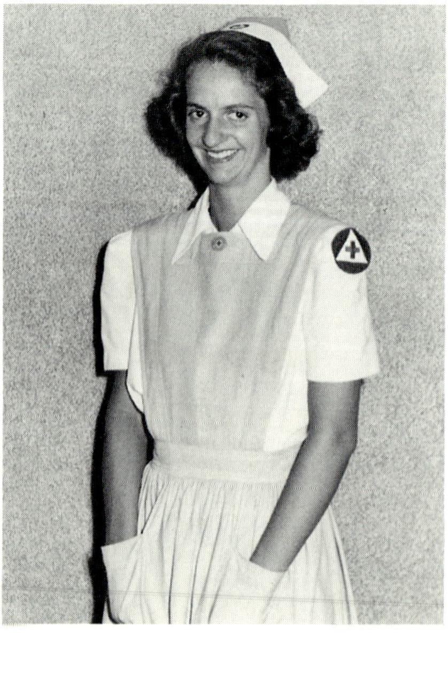

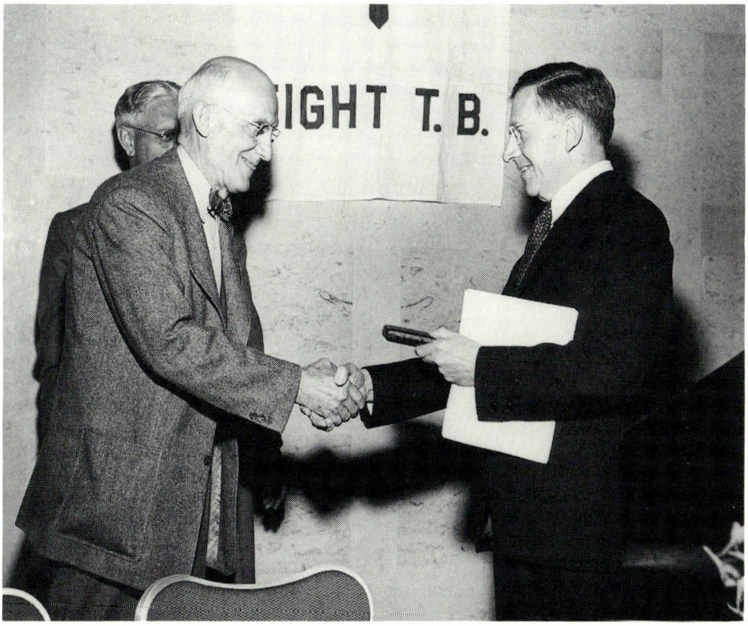

J. Burns Amberson, M.D., head of the chest service, Bellevue Hospital, New York City, presents the Trudeau Medal of the National Tuberculosis Association to his friend, James Waring, 1953.

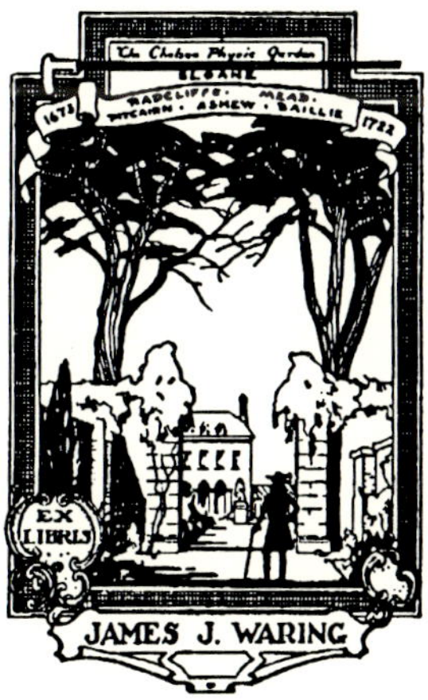

Waring's bookplate (see section on Gold-Headed Cane, pages 138-40)

Presented to the Library
University of Colorado
Medical Center, Denver

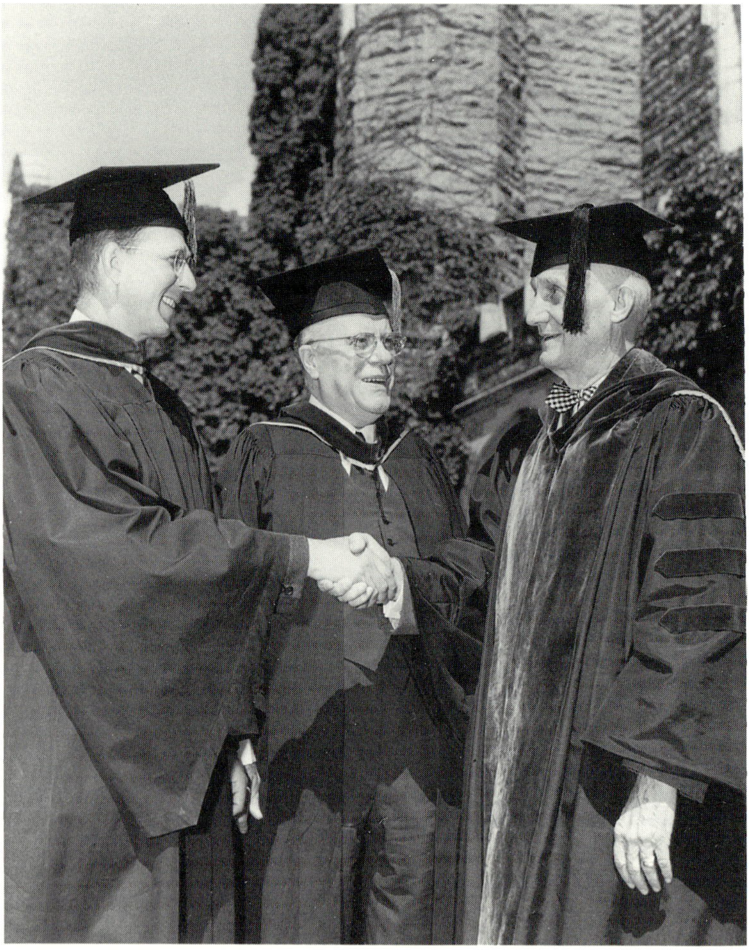

Waring (right) and Senator Eugene Millikin (middle), recipients of Norlin Medal for Distinguished Achievement at the University of Colorado commencement, June 9, 1951

part nonmedical, social organization. The founder of the club was Harold S. Walker, who had married Ruth's sister Laurene. Members shared meals in their club and gave papers on a great variety of subjects in an atmosphere both intellectual and congenial. After the mid-1930s a large unabridged dictionary was hung from the ceiling by an ingenious system devised by a member who was an engineer. Robert Stearns later reminisced about Waring's contributions to "literary discourses at the Cactus Club on the microscopic skills of Leeuwenhoek, the great Dutch naturalist, or his salty comments on Samuel Pepys on being 'cut for the stone'" (meaning Pepys would have had kidney stones removed, in that day a very painful procedure, usually involving removing the stones through the bladder, with no anesthetic).

Ruth appreciated her husband's enjoyment of these friendships, the relaxation of The Farm, whatever gave him pleasure. "She was very strong, very self-disciplined," says neighbor Polly Plesset. "They worked together. She had administrative skill, provided a well-run household.

"They were both very much in love. I went there often. Dr. Waring always gave her orchids for Christmas. I always thought they were romantic."

IN ONE CASE, Waring's forceful speaking of his mind led to a lawsuit. It happened this way: In 1933 an old friend at the Johns Hopkins School of Medicine, Dr. Edwards A. Park, wrote to say that Dr. Edgar A. Peterson, formerly of Denver and then working for a Ph.D. in chemistry at Hopkins, claimed to have discovered a drug to cure tuberculosis. Peterson was asking the cooperation of medical school doctors in getting permission to treat a large number of cases in an independent hospital, under the observation of other physicians, to demonstrate his formula.

The friendship of Drs. Park and Waring went back several years. Over a decade before, the latter wrote his wife that he had "poured out my woes to [Dr. Park] about the Children's Hospital and the medical school and got some sound advice." Now he had some advice of his own for Park:

> Dr. Peterson, the man about whom you make enquiries in your letter of February 9, is a thoroughly discredited person in this community. He has been guilty of serious malpractice and is a person for whom I have the utmost contempt and I have no hesitance in saying so. I would not trust him as far as I could throw a buffalo by the tail.[22] You can be sure I would not make this statement without ample ground for so doing.

> He has for years peddled his specific cure for tuberculosis in this town, telling all and sundry he has an absolute cure for tuberculosis. It has been a "secret remedy" and he has never published any statistics as to its use. He has tried to get some of the institutions in town to try his medicine, but all of them, knowing his reputation, have refused to do so.
>
> I think it would be a serious mistake to recognize him even to the extent of giving his remedy a trial. I have no doubt he would advertise thoroughly the fact that Johns Hopkins is trying his remedy and hope thereby to commercialize the prestige he could get from such a notice.

Park failed to keep Waring's letter confidential, and it fell into the hands of Peterson, who then filed a $250,000 libel suit in Denver District Court against Waring. Waring did not regret one word of his letter, but the suit would prove time-consuming, expensive, and emotionally exhausting. Although Peterson had a very poor reputation in Denver, evidence had to be shown to prove it. Seven Denver physicians, including Waring, gathered evidence of malpractice on the part of Peterson and submitted it to the Board of Censors of the Denver Medical Society. Some flagrant examples were presented, the worst being that of an eight-year old girl whose arm had to be amputated because Peterson had put it into a splint that was too tight, causing the child great pain and resulting in gangrene.

In another case, Peterson operated on a patient, not once but twice, for acute appendicitis. After the second operation the patient died, and a post-mortem examination showed that he had really been suffering from a perforated gastric ulcer, which Peterson had not detected. In still another case, Peterson had operated in a hospital with unsterilized instruments and had been forbidden by the superintendent ever to return.

But medical outrages were not Peterson's only failing. In the case of the patient who died after the second operation for appendicitis, Peterson had undertaken to rewrite the patient's will as he lay dying, naming himself as guardian of the children and executor of the estate. After the patient's death, Peterson sought to take possession of the estate. He lodged the will in the County Court of Denver, but it was never recognized. Some three years after bungling the case of the little girl's broken arm, Peterson went to Dallas and represented himself as an orthopedic surgeon.

As for his secret cure, Peterson claimed that it would remedy not only tuberculosis but also osteomyelitis, cancer, sinus colds, influenza, pneumonia, eye infections, boils and carbuncles, arthritis, and appendicitis. He steadfastly refused to reveal his formula's contents, although once or twice he hinted it contained mercury.

Waring's lawyers, Van Cise and Robinson, filed a request for documentary evidence from Peterson, including the formula for his cure and all records of experiments with it. Peterson's attorney then offered to drop the case if Waring would write to Johns Hopkins and say he was not opposed to Peterson's conducting experiments there. Waring refused, and the suit was dismissed, at Peterson's cost, upon motion of his attorney; this was even before the evidence of malpractice had been collected. Waring had won, but he sustained $5,000 in legal expenses.

In January 1936 another letter arrived from Park; Peterson was still at Johns Hopkins, still working on his Ph.D. and still blaming "a powerful person in Denver" as the cause of his troubles. One of the professors in the Johns Hopkins chemistry department was impressed with Peterson, considered him "a genius," and was in favor of granting him a Ph.D. The professor had told Park that he did not believe any of the charges brought against Peterson except "insofar as they involve errors in judgment or conduct that any one of us might make." Waring replied confidentially that he wanted to avoid any further controversy involving Peterson. He said that "Mrs. Waring is convinced that for me to take part actively in preventing this man from getting his Ph.D. degree would be for me to display a hostility toward him that might lead many to believe that I was really persecuting him." He referred Park to the other Denver doctors who had complained of Peterson's various malpractices.

And so an end came to the Peterson case. As a postscript, among Waring's memorabilia was a yellowed clipping, undated, from the *Baltimore Sun.* The story told of Dr. Edgar A. Peterson, "who was burned to death Saturday night at his home." Peterson, "a well-known authority and research worker on arthritis remedies," had for more than twenty years been working on intravenous injections as a cure for arthritis. He was working on a new arthritis serum in a laboratory in his home at the time of his death, when he apparently fell asleep while smoking a cigarette.

WHAT BEGAN in young James Waring as an interest in books became a passion in the man. "Love of good books is contagious and can be acquired readily. I have a prescription for its acquisition," he said in a talk to medical students. "All it needs is an inquiring mind, an eager concern to get knowledge, a quality indispensable in a doctor, anyhow." In a form requested by the Yale-Sheffield class of 1904 on its twenty-fifth anniversary, he wrote, "I have a very valuable collection of books relating to tuberculosis and diseases of the chest, which are my special interest." Widely read in the classics, he also enjoyed books on the American West and appreciated poetry. When Houstoun Waring, as a young man, told his older cousin that he liked the poetry of Robert W. Service, the doctor "blew his stack"; he thought Houstoun should set his sights higher.

Waring's particular area of expertise was medical history. With his near reverence for such figures as Laënnec, he spread his enthusiasm for the great medical figures of the past in his teaching and his medical papers. He volunteered his services as medical librarian to the library of the Denver Medical Society because he believed it important that the society have a good collection. A permanent medical library endowment fund had been started in 1912 following the merger of the University of Colorado College of Medicine and the faculty of the Denver and Gross Medical College. Before Waring's arrival in Denver, Dr. Charles Spivak had begun acquiring books and journals for the medical community. The library was at that time located in the Metropolitan Building, which is where Waring had his office.

At some point his love of reading turned into a love of collecting, probably around 1918. A decade later Allen Krause, a fellow student at Hopkins, sent him bookplates, letters, a pen-and-ink sketch and some autographed letters from H. L. Mencken. Far from collecting items of only medical historical importance, Waring amassed a wide variety of books and folios. The works of John James Audubon, artist and naturalist, and Izaak Walton, author in the seventeenth century of *The Compleat Angler,* were among his favorites. "I also have a very valuable collection of Waltonia—every fisherman will know what that means," he wrote on the form requested by the Yale class of 1904.

He grew up in a home where books were highly valued. His great-grandfather, who bequeathed his library of several hundred books to the first of his sons who should study the profession of medicine, had said, "I will and direct that no expense shall be spared to give my children the very best education as I desire them to be well and thoroughly educated." Another element in collecting was the thrill of pursuit, of holding a book that had the handcrafted look of years past, the smell of another era. Waring knew the importance of a medical library to medical schools, but he also realized that its development meant seeking near and far to find essential volumes.

Perhaps the best known collector in the field was his mentor, William Osler, who left his collection to McGill University in Montreal. Waring visited the Osler collection and sent Ruth a postcard stating that the library "contains 7,000 volumes." Osler said: "A physician who does not need a library . . . soon sinks to the level of a cross-counter prescriber." Another famed medical scholar, Harvard lecturer Paul Dudley White, wrote, "Do not fill your library full of modern books and journals: leave plenty of space and money for the more important books of the past, dating back if possible to the time of the first printing presses." White thought it important to secure representative volumes of the sixteenth through nineteenth centuries: "A classic or a leading textbook of the past is far more valuable than a second-rate volume of the present."

It was James Waring's good fortune to be in a position to collect old volumes, but he was an inveterate bargain hunter and set a limit on how much he would spend, resisting the profligate, impulsive purchase. In a letter to Ruth in 1925, he commented on a bookseller in New York City: "I offended (?) him by telling him he had the reputation for charging unconscionable prices!! He said the Laënnecs were in great demand and very high priced and he had none for sale! I bought a first edition Austin Flint on 'Phthisis' 1878 for $7.50." A sales slip, dated April 16, 1926, is tucked inside Waring's copy of *Senensis Medici* by Andreae Matthioli, 1569. The bill of sale is from a London bookstore, showing that the doctor was even then ranging far afield in his quest for books.

Waring had a partner in his collecting, for Ruth encouraged her husband to indulge his passion. He seemed to take as much pleasure in donating books as he did in acquiring them; again, Ruth agreed. The pain of parting with his acquisitions had the advantage of leaving empty space on the shelves, thus giving him incentive to buy more. Both daughters remember how crowded the bookshelves were on all the floors of 910 Gaylord Street. Because books abounded, eventually Waring added a study and many stacks for books on the third floor and a small elevator so he would not have to go up the back stairs. The study was made more inviting by the addition of a large window looking toward the mountains, but the room was seldom used, for it was too far away from his family. He preferred reading in bed and having his wife nearby.

Browsing in rare-book stores held endless fascination for Waring, as did looking at catalogues. Corresponding with important dealers also was part of the hobby. He kept within the price limit he had set for himself, and his familiarity with medical history gave him a sharp eye for books in this field. If a dealer asked more than $100 for a book, his response was that he could not afford it.

A classmate at Johns Hopkins, Herbert M. Evans, also was an inveterate collector. An anatomist and endocrinologist and a discoverer of Vitamin E (in 1922 with K. S. Bishop), over the course of his life Evans began, then sold, at least seven collections in the history of medicine and science. In 1932, then holder of the Chair of Anatomy at the University of California, Evans wrote to Waring for help in finding a buyer. This was the first collection he would sell.

> Dear Jim, I hope you will find a donor for my collection of medical classics and history of medicine. It is like tearing my heart out to sell it but it simply must be done and I do not want to peddle it. I also wish to say that any sum you consider reasonable will likely be the selling price for I am sure I simply cannot get the value it will one day have. Ever since we graduated I have sunk from a thousand dollars up (some years two thousand) yearly in it and I really believe the hundred finest books (the great ones) are probably worth as much as ten thousand dollars alone. . . . You will note there are no comments on the importance of the books. . . . Perhaps the Vesalius, Jenner, and Withering and Asellius are the greatest single items.

Ruth Waring and her sister Dora offered to buy the collection and donate it to the Denver Medical Society library. The price was $18,000. Terms dictated that payment was to be made in installments over a period of years, ending in 1936. Although the sisters did pay the major portion of the asking price, there were other contributors as well, and, under an arrangement made in 1945, the Warings paid to the medical society library the amount that the others had contributed, with the donors' and board of trustees' approval.

The society had purchased some old medical texts in 1929 and was provided with funds for further purchases in the will of Dr. Walter Jayne. The addition of the Evans collection was a windfall: 850 bound volumes and 984 reprints. The anatomical classics were remarkably complete. Some of the treasures in the collection: a first edition, illustrated, of Vesalius of Padua's *De humani corporis fabrica,* 1543, and a second edition of the book, Basel 1555. The 1543 book reportedly was Evans's favorite in the collection, along with *China Root Epistle* of Vesalius, Basel, 1546.

With the acquisition of the Evans collection, James Waring's place among the brotherhood of collectors was recognized, and in 1934 he received a letter from the widow of Dr. LeRoy Crummer, a well-known collector: "I am anxiously awaiting the receipt of your sketch of Crummer as I am hoping to get the biography under way so I can go abroad this Fall." A correspondent wrote Waring: "Dr. LeRoy Crummer's library of rare medical books is considered one of the three finest medical libraries in the country. It includes 442 medical books printed before the year 1640."

Being a collector meant being part of a fellowship of like-minded people who helped each other—sometimes—in their quests. He had joined "a third class of men in the [medical] profession to whom books are dearer than to teachers or practitioners." Osler had described them in "Books and Men, in Dedication of the . . . Boston Medical Library" (1901) as "a small, a silent band, but in reality the leaven of the whole lump. . . . Loving books partly for their contents, partly for the sake of the authors. . . . We need more men of their class, particularly in this country, where every one carries in his pocket the tape measure of utility."

Dr. Harvey Cushing, pioneer neurosurgeon and biographer of Osler, went to Johns Hopkins for surgical training, and there his interest in collecting received direction from Osler, Welch, and Kelly. He acquired the 1543 first edition of Vesalius's *Fabrica,* and Kelly gave him the 1555 second edition. James Waring must have been delighted, in 1939, to learn that a letter from Cushing, a towering figure on the faculty at Hopkins when he was a student there, had arrived in the medical society's mail: "Dear Sirs, I am informed that you have an unusually fine copy of the *De humani corporis fabrica* formerly belonging to Herbert M. Evans. I will be greatly obliged if you will let me know what are the exact page dimensions of this copy. Sincerely yours, Harvey Cushing."[23]

There was another link with Cushing. Dr. Esmond R. Long, director of the Henry Phipps Institute at the University of Pennsylvania, received many books from Waring, much prized by him. Long, in turn, gave Waring a first edition of *The Gold-Headed Cane,* which he had received from Harvey Cushing. As collectors, they were bound by their enthusiasm for medical history.

Part Four | *Department Head*

8 | *Professor of Medicine*

A FAMILY VACATION in 1931 at Granite Peaks Camp, east of Durango Colorado, near Wolf Creek Pass, started out in high spirits. Uncle Antonio was there from Savannah with his family, joining James, Ruth, and the girls. Joking, teasing, and laughter accompanied these family reunions. What happened next came without warning.

"Daddy had a bow and arrow, and with the exertion of pulling back the bow, he pulled loose a lesion in his chest," his daughter Ruth explains. "He knew it—he knew his body so well that he knew he'd broken something loose. He went to bed for a year."

This was the sort of thing James Waring had long feared. In his paper "Relapse in Tuberculosis" (1923), he described the possible effects of overexertion. In this case, he may have suffered a spontaneous pneumothorax, in which air escapes into the pleural cavity as a result of injury of lung tissue. He knew the importance of moderation. Pinned to the frontispiece of *Daily Strength for Daily Needs,* which he kept by his bed—probably a gift from his mother, who kept a copy by her bed—was a dog-eared quotation, author unknown: "There are times when one must sacrifice his body in order to serve a higher end . . . but the general law of health is this: You have no more right to over-drive it in your ambition until it breaks down, than you would overwork your servant or over-drive your horse."

But there was no sense in regretting what had happened. He turned adversity to advantage and used his time well, reading prodigiously. He began editing a column in *Colorado Medicine* entitled "Library Notes," writing on such diverse subjects as "Three Doctors of the French Revolution" and on the fiftieth anniversary of Robert Koch's discovery of the tubercle bacillus. Writing this column was providential for him during this time of recuperation, providing a forum in which to share his interest in the history of medicine.

He wrote papers, including three concerning high altitude, but foremost among his projects was writing "The History of Artificial Pneumothorax," a paper on the chief treatment for tuberculosis at that time. Researching the subject was no small undertaking. Among his effects are nine legal-sized pads of references. His correspondence was international. In all, he spent three years gathering and compiling the material. *The Journal of the Outdoor Life* of the National Tuberculosis Association published the book-length manuscript in five installments from September 1933 through January 1934. An announcement appearing in the *New England Journal of Medicine* stated that "the series is by a well-known physician. . . . The comparatively recent rise of surgery in the treatment of tuberculosis has focused the attention of both tuberculosis specialists and of general surgeons on this method."

In these days of computer searches, when librarians are able to produce extensive bibliographies within minutes, the barriers placed in Waring's path seem formidable. Locating relevant literature often was difficult, as when he was advised by several Italian sources that the only copies of a privately printed booklet, *Rivista,* by Dr. Carlo Forlanini—a pioneer in the procedure—were unavailable because they were in private hands. A correspondent from R. Lier & Company, antiquarian booksellers in Florence, Italy, wrote: "We have written in the last two months more than 25 letters. Although having excellent relations to the most prominent Italian physicians, universities, etc., we have not been able to trace a copy of this *Rivista*. . . . Forlanini's brother . . . writes us, as follows: 'Myself, I have one single copy and I have not at all the intention to sell it.' Therefore it will be probably impossible to find a copy."

Apparently Waring *did* obtain a copy: A cryptic note pencilled on the letter says "Coolidge St. Paul," so possibly the sought-after Rivista came from a U.S. source. The medical library resources of Denver were limited, so he enlisted some help in tracing references from one Harriet Blogg, who seems to have been connected with the Johns Hopkins medical school. In addition, he asked the help of librarians at the Osler Library at McGill, the Crerar Medical Library in Chicago, the New York Academy of Medicine, and the Institute of the History of Medicine. For translation of the Italian, primarily in the articles by and about Dr. Carlo Forlanini, he relied upon a Dr. Albi of Denver—presumably Dr. Piero Albi, who spoke and wrote Italian and whose father, Dr. Rudolph Albi, had come to Denver at the turn of the century from Italy, where he had been a professor of surgery in Milan.

The several typewritten drafts of the paper, with Waring's changes, indicate the care with which he revised his work, taking into account new information and always seeking precise wording. No indication is given as to who read the manuscript, but Gerald Webb may have assisted. It was he who introduced artificial pneumothorax to the Rocky

Mountain region in 1912 after attending a meeting in Rome at which Forlanini's accomplishment was discussed.

In the introduction Waring told of his reservations regarding the use of the procedure, then controversial and now discredited, in which the diseased lung is collapsed by introducing gas or air into the chest cavity. "Satisfactory as is the use of artificial pneumothorax, marvelous as are its results sometimes in speed and completeness, still would it be unwise to say either that this method has come to stay or that with the passage of time it would undergo no modification in technique or application."

In his chronology he went back to the fourth century B.C. to "the Hippocratic physician [who] treated adhesive pleuritis secondary to a wound or empyema [pus in a bodily cavity] by sending air into the interior of the chest through the accidental wound in the chest wall or through the operative wound for empyema drainage." He credited Laënnec, ever his medical hero, with being "the first to recognize pneumothorax in the living subject" (1819) and cited Dr. Daniel McRuer, who practiced medicine in Bangor, Maine, for recommending puncture of the chest to suspend the action of a diseased lung (1835). To his old friend Lawrason Brown of Saranac Lake he gave credit "for unearthing this historical note."

To whom should go the credit for first performing the procedure? "An unfortunate controversy as to priority was precipitated," he wrote. He gave Forlanini credit for "inspiration, quiet meditation." Dr. John Murphy of the United States came later and made his discovery "independently as a result of shrewd and clinical observation."

What were the objections to the treatment? He cited the risk of losing a useful lung. If immobilization is good for one lung, why would overwork be good for the other? He expressed the view of the internist: "Enthusiasm for surgical collapse has on occasion elbowed the man with the stethoscope away from his position of leadership at the bedside and replaced him with a surgeon. Treatment has become social, surgical, institutional, governmental, and no longer remains predominately personal, climatic and medical." But in conclusion he maintained an open mind on the procedure: "Suddenly, about 1912 America woke up and before the lapse of another three years nearly every Sanatorium in the country . . . was using it. Today artificial pneumothorax is a well-tried and proven procedure of incalculable benefit in properly selected cases."

Letters from all over the United States and from abroad poured into Waring's office at 203 Metropolitan Building. The controversy concerned who was the first to perform artificial pneumothorax. Dr. G. Walter Holden of Denver, who had been director of the Agnes Phipps Memorial Sanitarium at the time Waring worked there twenty years before, wrote on September 27, 1933: "I performed the first artificial collapse of a tuberculous lung in Denver . . . in 1909." A letter in English from Edouard Rist, M.D., advised that Dr. Dumarest was the first and that he was the third to employ the operation in France. Lawrason Brown, his old friend, wrote that the first case tried in Saranac Lake "was done by me in 1912."

Of particular interest, in view of the number of doctors who wrote to Waring saying they were among the first to use the operation, is that one doctor shunned attention. Several medical men had written to Waring regarding Dr. Mary Lapham of Highlands, North Carolina. "Read her renowned paper before the national [meeting]—I think in 1912—on artificial pneumothorax," wrote one. "Lapham was the first to give [pneumothorax] wide publicity," pointed out another.

Lapham wrote to Waring, July 27, 1932: "As soon as a paper of mine was accepted, I forgot all about it and have never kept a record of any of them so that I do not know what or when I have written. From memory I should say that they were all of very little account and not worth mentioning, so that it wouldn't matter a bit whether they were or were not included in your list." Among Waring's memorabilia is a picture of the self-effacing Lapham, dressed in what appears to be an Army uniform topped by an atrocious hat.

Waring discussed her contributions in his paper and compiled a bibliography of her writings on the subject. "In 1912," he wrote, "the joint paper by Hamman and Sloan and that of Mary E. Lapham of North Carolina were the first papers on pneumothorax to be read before the National Association for the Study and Prevention of Tuberculosis. Indeed Mary Lapham, who learned the technique in 1909 from von Muralt at Davos-Dorf, Switzerland, deserves much of the credit for bringing to the attention of American physicians this most useful procedure. Between 1910 and 1913 she published nine reports of her experience with pneumothorax."

Not only did he give credit where it was due to these three; in Lewis Hamman's case, he also paid tribute to the Johns Hopkins professor who told Gerald Webb that Jim Waring was "the most promising medical student" he had seen. As for Mary Lapham, he recognized a modest physician who had wrongly dismissed her papers as being "all of very little account."

Originally the editor of *The Journal of the Outdoor Life* indicated that the first of the series would appear in March 1933, but Waring had not finished. In May 1933 he was back at Johns Hopkins for a checkup. "Have same room as I had when I was taken sick as student here 27 years ago last month," he wrote Ruth. It also gave him an opportunity to use the Johns Hopkins library as he raced the clock to finish the series. He wrote Ruth on May 15: "The library here is magnificent and am putting in some worthwhile licks on the pneumothorax history." In September the first article appeared.

Waring had good reason to be in such a rush to finish the paper, quite apart from the journal's deadline. This was the year he became the first full-time head of the Department of Medicine, as well as professor of medicine, at the University of Colorado School of Medicine. Lewis Hamman would have been proud.

BY 1931, when James Waring had to withdraw from the medical school's volunteer faculty because of illness, his effectiveness as a teacher and diagnostician and his reputation as a scholar were well recognized. Dean Maurice Rees was aware of his gifts; thus when Dr. Charles N. Meader resigned as head of the Department of Medicine in 1932, it was recommended to the Board of Regents that Waring be named to replace him. On June 15, 1933, the faculty voted to accept "the appointment of Dr. James J. Waring to the Professorship in Medicine and Head of the Department." With the concurrence of the regents, it was now official.

Dean Rees wrote to President O. C. Lester of the University of Colorado, on June 16, 1933: "I feel quite sure that Dr. Waring will be willing to devote the major portion of his time to the work of the department, since he has indicated that given this position, he would be willing to give up most of his practice. Dr. Waring is a recognized authority on tuberculosis . . . and is one of the best teachers we have had in the School of Medicine."

James Waring thus became the first full-time professor of medicine to head the Department of Medicine at the University of Colorado medical school. (Julius Wilson, M.D., who succeeded Esmond Long as director of the Henry Phipps Institute of the University of Pennsylvania, wrote that James Waring was the first specialist in tuberculosis to become a full-time professor and head of a department of medicine.) He was not paid by the university for his services for well over a decade. It was agreed that he would retain some private patients when he assumed his duties; but even so, without his wife's support, it would have been difficult for him to accept the dual appointment.

Why was he not paid for so long? It was not unusual at that time for clinical faculty to serve without pay. Furthermore, the medical school was in poor financial shape because of the Depression, which had gripped the nation following the 1929 stock market crash. Finances for the medical school in 1933 were in such straits that it was feared that both Colorado General and Colorado Psychopathic hospitals might have to close.

On top of the funding problem, there was opposition from doctors in private practice who believed that full-time clinical faculty should receive only fees for consultations, not for routine care. The controversy over "full-time" faculty was more complicated than merely "Town vs. Gown." Only one other full-time clinical faculty member served in the medical school, Franklin Ebaugh, professor in psychiatry and head of that department since 1925. In 1924 a letter from Rees to Ebaugh showed the curious ambivalence within the academic community about full-time work:

> Our attitude on the question of outside consultation work by full-time members of the faculty is that such members must be responsible primarily for the conduct of teaching, clinical and executive work attendant on their position . . . but that having satisfied such obligations, the University interposes no objection to a man doing as much outside consultation work as he can conscientiously. . . . Regarding the acquisition of such outside consultation practice as an indirect asset to the University[,] . . . a strictly full-time position without outside contact tends to rapidly institutionalize a man and thus diminish the breadth of view desirable in a teaching position. . . . [Therefore, we believe] that contact in the right way with practicing physicians in the city and state by members of the University tends to strengthen their interest in the University and their support, and that affording expert professional service to the practicing physicians of the state through them to its people is one of the broader functions of the University.

The controversy was not new. Victor O. Freeburg in *William Henry Welch at Eighty* stated that when Welch said that Hopkins would initiate full-time positions, Osler, who had become Regius Professor at Oxford University, said publicly in disgust that full-time teaching would probably lead to the production of "a set of clinical prigs, the boundary of whose horizon would be the laboratory, and whose only human interest would be research." But by the 1930s, progressive schools gravitated toward full-time faculty, as did Osler toward the end of his life.

In his new capacity, Waring regarded his primary missions as training physicians and providing excellent patient care. He had inherited a variety of challenges, including the lack of adequate funding and the need for more faculty members in order to replace the old lecture system of teaching with that of clinical and bedside instruction. The bright side of his chairmanship was that he was able to recruit some outstanding doctors, all practicing physicians who volunteered their time to the hospital and the clinics without financial recompense.

Dr. Ward Darley was promoted from assistant outpatient physician to outpatient physician. A graduate of the medical school's class of 1929, he was seen as having marked ability. Dr. Vera Heinly Jones received a similar appointment, and in October, Dr. Anna Grace Seyler was among three doctors appointed assistant outpatient physician. Now two women were on Waring's service at a time when there were few female medical school graduates.

Dr. Robert S. Liggett was appointed assistant in medicine, Outpatient Department, to begin July 1, 1935. Born in 1903 in St. Louis, Liggett received a degree from the Washington University School of Medicine in 1933. He served a medical residency at Colorado General Hospital from 1934 to 1935 and apparently impressed Waring, for they joined in private practice soon after Liggett's residency and became close friends. "A very good combination" is the assessment of Dr. Charles Freed, who served as a resident at about this time.

At the 1963 Waring symposium, Liggett told of their close friendship: "Jim always felt toward me like a father toward a son, and I always felt toward him like a son toward a father. I am happy to say that at no time in our twenty-five or more years of association did we ever have any serious differences. We enjoyed practicing together."

Other appointments of note were Dr. Abe Ravin to instructor in medicine, and promotions for Drs. Thaddeus Sears and Dumont Clark in 1935. Waring's recommendation that Dr. Charles Kaufman of the National Jewish Hospital be offered an assistant professorship in medicine (tuberculosis) helped strengthen the ties between the two institutions.

It was James Waring who put forth the idea, adopted in 1929, of having Gerald Webb lecture on the history of medicine at the medical school. The two friends enjoyed their weekly luncheons together. When Webb was unable to continue his teaching, Dr. Nolie Mumey, who was well qualified to teach this subject, was appointed lecturer in medicine.

One of the teaching tools of a medical school is grand rounds, the name given to the general faculty meeting. In the 1930s they were held in the evening; attendance varied. The largest audience shown in the Executive Faculty Minutes in that decade appears to be ninety-five, when Waring and a colleague discussed "Dissecting Aneurysm of the Aorta" on April 11, 1938. The variety of cases Waring was given to discuss shows the breadth of knowledge the professor of medicine was expected to have: carcinoma of the pancreas; myasthenia gravis; cavitary pulmonary tuberculosis (discussion also with Dr. R. W. Arndt); massive pyo-pneumothorax following bronchiectasis (with Dr. Charles J. Lowen); visceral syphilis; carcinoma of the lung; metastasis from teratoma of testis; thrombo-angitis obliterans (with Dr. Frank B. Queen).

The head of medicine also sat on many medical school committees. In one of Waring's notebooks, in his handwriting, is this pithy comment: "Committees keep minutes but waste hours!" Within three months of taking on his new position he had been made chairman of a special committee on isolation technique on the wards, followed a few months later by the chairmanship of an advisory committee to the Social Service Department. Three more committee assignments followed in 1934. And so it went. In 1937 Dean Rees appointed him chairman of a committee to prepare a form for taking a patient's medical history, a subject of particular concern to Waring, who had always taken a keen interest in this vital part of patient care.

Since 1927 Waring and other faculty members had been working to change instruction in the medical school from large class to individual student sessions, and by the mid-1930s he had influenced others to this point of view. But the old lecture system was slow to change. In 1936 the medical school was inspected and evaluated by a committee responsible to the Council on Medical Education and Hospitals of the American Medical Association, chaired by Dean Weiskotten from Syracuse University Medical School. Lowest in its rating was the Department of Medicine. As related in *The University of Colorado School of Medicine: A Centennial History* by Dr. Robert H. Shikes and Dr. Henry N. Claman, "The committee felt that, except for Waring: 'The clinical men were not familiar with the work being done in their departments, and . . . allowed courses to spring up which had no connection with the coordinated course.'" Too many lectures, not enough time at the bedside for the students.

The evaluating committee recommended that the school employ two to three full-time clinical men to help coordinate clinical teaching, and therein lay a problem. The state's coffers were greatly depleted because of the financial havoc caused by the Depression. Since the late

1920s, the state legislature had enacted a permanent mill levy that went toward maintenance, but a shortage of funds persisted. Dean Rees sought aid from the Rockefeller Foundation in 1938 for support of full-time paid members on the staffs of the clinical departments, but the foundation did not lend its support this time as it had with the building program of the 1920s (see Chapter 5).

In July 1936 Henry Sewall died. He had remained active in his eighties, grateful to National Jewish Hospital for providing him space in which to continue his work. Mrs. Sewall (or perhaps Sewall before his death) gave Waring several of Sewall's letters from distinguished correspondents as diverse as Wilfred Grenfell and H. L. Mencken. James Waring made arrangements for a memorial meeting for Sewall at the Brown Palace, giving a biographical sketch with lantern slides. A Sewall lectureship was established. Among Waring's papers is a bill from the Denver Country Club for a party in 1954 for fifty-one guests, with the notation, "Sewall lecture."

Besides remaining active in the Denver Medical Society, serving on three committees from 1931 to 1937, Waring was a delegate to the Colorado Medical Society from 1934 to 1936. Despite having limited energy, he also was becoming more involved in national organizations, taking on the presidency of the National Tuberculosis Association from 1935 to 1936. In 1938 he became a governor of the American College of Physicians, a society of doctors specializing in internal medicine and related specialties. Waring's participation in professional organizations reflected a desire to continually sharpen his expertise. Quoting Osler in the Cushing biography on the need for reverberation of ideas among colleagues: "No class of men needs friction so much as physicians; no class gets less. The daily round of a busy practitioner tends to develop an egoism of a most intense kind, to which there is no antidote. The few setbacks are forgotten, the mistakes are often buried. . . . To this mental attitude the medical society is the best corrective, and a man misses a good part of his education who does not get knocked about a bit by his colleagues in discussions and criticisms."

Waring's penchant for self-criticism came through in a letter to Ruth in May 1933; he had just given a speech in Washington, D.C., and felt it "a sad failure." He was oppressed with the thought that everybody was weary. "I tried to cut it and in so doing destroyed its continuity—which was just too bad!!!" In another letter to Ruth in the 1930s, he wrote of wanting to "learn new things, meet new people." He liked the interchange; he also liked the camaraderie. He became known as a man of humor and charm, who, in the words of a colleague, "could step up the morale of any dull session of meetings with telling witty stories." He also liked a friendly card game between sessions.

Waring continued his affiliation with the Colorado Foundation for Research in Tuberculosis. As vacancies occurred on the advisory council in the mid-1930s, the places were taken by Drs. Esmond R. Long and Florence R. Sabin. Long, a pathologist and director of the Henry Phipps Institute at the University of Pennsylvania, was another former patient at Saranac Lake and longtime friend of Waring. Sabin was the first woman to graduate from the Johns Hopkins School of Medicine; the first woman to intern at Hopkins; and the first woman to teach in the Hopkins medical school. As an instructor of freshmen in anatomy, she probably taught Waring in that subject. She was the first female faculty member at Hopkins to become a full professor, then left teaching in 1925 to join the Rockefeller Institute for Medical Research in New York, heading the Department of Cellular Studies, and coordinated studies on tuberculosis in various institutions. With retirement mandatory at sixty-five, she returned to Denver in the late 1930s to live with her sister, a fortuitous move for her home state. She and James Waring would become friends, working for many of the same causes.

Of James Waring's papers written in the 1930s, one stands out alongside his magnum opus on artificial pneumothorax: "The Vicissitudes of Auscultation" (1936). This paper in support of the stethoscope, now considered a classic, was his address as president of the National Tuberculosis Association. It was a subject he approached with enthusiasm, for in it he lauded his hero, Laënnec:

> Three francs put Laënnec's wooden, monaural stethoscope in the hands of the doctor. Three dollars puts the modern instrument in the hands of the medical student. Dwell on this instrument a moment more. Its initial cost is trivial, its maintenance and depreciation charges are not worth mentioning, it does not require an extra room at fifty dollars per month rental to house it, and no extra charge is made to the patient if it proves necessary to use it. It is portable, excessively convenient, almost indestructible. Although some doctors neglect it or use it carelessly, it richly rewards the man who uses it painstakingly.

Laënnec received respect but no enthusiasm for his invention. By 1826, when he died, wrote Waring, "practically every stethoscope in existence was the product of his own hand." Samuel George Morton studied with Laënnec and brought his method back to the United States.

William Waring, James Waring's nephew and Jane B. Aron Professor of Pediatrics, Tulane School of Medicine, spent some time in Japan in the Army Medical Corps. In 1985, when he attended the International Lung Sounds Conference in Tokyo, Dr. Shoji Judoh presented him with a copy of a talk Judoh had given in 1936, quoting James Waring's paper. At the top of the paper, in English, Judoh quoted the concluding paragraph of "The Vicissitudes of Auscultation," including the same paragraph in Japanese at the bottom of the paper:

> In conclusion: Are centuries of bedside experience assembled by thousands of observers to be tossed to oblivion while we chase the will-o'-the wisp of the X ray through the unreal land of lights and shadows? The answer is: No! The history of physical diagnosis teaches us that nothing good is ever lost. Auscultation increased the value of percussion; roentgenography increases the value of both. Let the slogan of the stethoscopist be: Listen, look and listen again.

A letter of January 19, 1938, from Dean Maurice Rees to President George Norlin tells of a dispute between Waring and Dr. Clough T. Burnett, an associate professor in the Department of Medicine and head of electrocardiography. Apparently Waring thought his associate was "calling from the ward more patients than he could possibly use for his own class work."

> Dean Rees:
> It has been my impression that Dr. Burnett is attempting to make things as unpleasant for Dr. Waring as possible. . . . I agree that both . . . are highly temperamental, but it has been my feeling right along that Dr. Burnett was the principal aggressor, and that if he were only willing to be more agreeable and more willing to cooperate with Dr. Waring, there would be no further difficulty. Dr. Waring assured me this morning that he would see to it that Dr. Burnett always had sufficient material for his class work.

Hardly a first-class feud, it was more of a tempest in a teapot. Dr. Charles Freed recalls that friction existed between "two of the general surgeons and the internists." Waring, in his gracious manner, usually won the battle."[24]

Occasional conflict was unavoidable for one so outspoken. Never afraid to express his opinion, Waring thought others also should be allowed to do so. Years later, Robert Liggett, his partner in private practice, told the Waring symposium about a Denver Medical Society meeting at which motions were made to censor the members of the society who had subscribed to the idea of socialized medicine. "Jim got up and made the most beautiful speech that I've ever heard about one's right to express his opinion. . . . In closing he said, 'When the time comes that a man cannot express an opinion, then it's time to get the old musket down off the fireplace.' He . . . wouldn't be censored by a bunch of individuals who had nothing to offer but small talk, and Jim was too big for that."

As the 1930s ended, the roller coaster cycle of inadequate funding led Dean Rees to inform President Norlin that, without a supplemental appropriation, the medical school would have to suspend operations. Government grants in 1939 helped. Despite financial problems, the medical school was making progress and would be greatly put to the test in the years just ahead.

James Waring always had been a hard worker. Taking over the department at almost fifty, following one of three extended periods of bed rest while recuperating from his most recent flare-up of illness, he had worked harder than ever, somehow finding hidden reserves of physical energy. Observe Shikes and Claman in *A Centennial History:* "Waring was undoubtedly the driving force in the clinical departments before World War II." He did not take lightly his responsibilities as a teacher, setting high objectives for his students and for himself. He agreed with William Osler's simple words: "I desire no other epitaph than the statement that I taught medical students in the wards, as I regard this as by far the most useful and important work I have been called upon to do."

IN THE 1930s, Annie Waring developed Parkinson's disease, for which there was then no treatment. She was lovingly cared for during many months of illness by Minna. On February 23, 1936, she died at the age of seventy-eight. Ruth happened to be away at the time with daughter Ruth; and Anne, then eleven, remembers that her father talked to her until late into the night about what an extraordinary woman his mother had been and how much he had loved her.

Her death was not unexpected. Six years earlier she had written:

"My beloved Tono and Jim: Look after your Aunt Minna—give her help and advice she may need and comfort and a home." Annie signed her will in 1932, leaving most of her possessions to Minna. The remainder was divided equally between Tono and Jim: "My Bible for Jim. My *Daily Strength for Daily Needs* for Antonio to use." Also specified was a sentimental bequest for each daughter-in-law and grandchild. After her death, James and Ruth donated to St. Barnabas Church in her memory a stained-glass window, to be designed by Charles J. Connick of Boston.

Another death in the family occurred the following year: Henry Porter died on July 25, 1937, at the age of ninety-eight. He had kept busy writing books in his later years. In accordance with his belief that "the man who dies rich dies disgraced," he had given away the greater part of his fortune and perhaps did not consider the remainder sufficient to classify himself as rich. Much of his philanthropy characteristically had been anonymous, as when, during the depression, he had trainloads of food distributed in Denver. On the day following his death, *The Denver Post* said of him: "What Denver is today is largely the result of the faith of men like Henry M. Porter. No showoffs, they, but strong, reliable, fearless, loyal citizens."

That autumn the Warings' daughter Ruth went away to school, enrolling in Mount Vernon Seminary, formerly Miss Summers's School (her mother's alma mater). Anne followed Ruth there the following year, and when Anne was going to New York City for a visit in November, her mother sent her a packet of postcards with the following message: "Before you go please stamp and address postcards to us and be sure to send us some sort of message every day and let us know definitely when you are going, where you are going and when you are returning to Washington." When, on occasion, Waring went to Washington or was passing through on medical business, he saw his daughters. In 1940 Anne wrote him, thanking him "for giving us a grand time in Washington, D.C. Daddy, I love you so much! I must study now."

His health was better now. There apparently was no recurrence of the colitis that had been a sporadic problem in the 1920s and perhaps as late as the 1930s. However, hay fever was a continual concern to him, especially in May and June. In the early 1930s he had a flare-up and went to Colorado Springs to see Drs. Gerald Webb and William Service, who were interested in allergies. Waring had difficulty in exhaling, and Service thought he might be suffering from asthma. He was checked on pollens and foods, this at a time when few people were doing such studies. He recovered well and was able to go back to work.

The Colorado Springs doctors were taking the first steps in using protein extract for testing allergies, and Waring was interested.

Fishing increasingly became his favorite diversion. Using dry fly fishing as a lure, he brought to Colorado a series of distinguished medical experts to speak at the medical school. Ruth was a willing hostess for the small but steady stream of guests that passed through over the years, debarking from a stopover in Colorado while on a transcontinental train trip.

Ruth had her own coterie of friends as well. In the 1930s she began playing bridge every Monday with Cyrena Toll, Alice McWhinney, and Eleanor Emery. They played regularly for forty years and became known as "The Homeless Women"—not to be confused with "The Loose Ladies," another group of friends who dined together. At the beginning of each year for a month or two, McWhinney recalls, Ruth could not play bridge because she was spending so much time on bookkeeping.

Ruth also generously supported various philanthropies, but she saved her most important support for her husband. In the latter half of the 1930s, she backed him up in his innovative leap into research. Waring was going to introduce a new division into the Department of Medicine, one that would require her financial backing.

Earlier in the 1930s, Waring had become interested in industrial hygiene, also known as industrial medicine (today referred to as "occupational health"). Interest in occupational health dates back to the Greeks and Romans; Hippocrates, in the fourth century B.C., recognized the toxic properties of lead. In the twentieth century progress was made, particularly in Great Britain and Germany, with regulation of trades injurious to health, but the United States lagged behind. The U.S. Bureau of Mines began investigating hygienic and safety conditions in mines,[25] and because a good deal of mining was done in Colorado, this was the industry in which Waring was most interested.

In 1936 the government appointed four committees "to head a cooperative campaign to lessen the ravages of the disease to which a half-million workers were said to be exposed." The American Medical Association that year recommended that every state medical society should have "an active committee devoted to the study of the problems of industrial medicine."[26]

The first hint of a new Division of Industrial Hygiene at the University of Colorado School of Medicine appears in the Executive Faculty Minutes of April 5, 1937: "On the recommendation of Dr. James Waring motion was made that Mr. Donald E. Cummings be appointed Fellow in Medicine." The first direct mention in the minutes came on August 14,

1939: "James Waring presented a proposition of establishing a Division of Industrial Hygiene in the Department of Medicine to be financed by funds received by Dr. Waring from private sources and guaranteed for a period of five years. . . . Also, that Mr. Donald E. Cummings be appointed associate professor of medicine and director of Division of Industrial Hygiene." An industrial hygienist with a degree in chemical engineering, Cummings went to Saranac Lake after developing tuberculosis. He became a consultant on dust control to the mining industry and assistant director of the Saranac Laboratory, which is where he met Waring.

Waring made himself personally responsible for raising about $10,000 a year for the support of the new division, the first within the department. The program was initially supported by Dora Porter Mason (Ruth's sister), Mary Dean Reed, the Boettcher Foundation, and Ruth Waring. In 1942 Reed made another significant contribution. James Waring also sought backing from industry. He probably was influenced by the Metropolitan Life Insurance Company's Framingham experiment, called "the first real attempt at comprehensive community hygiene in the United States." Climax Molybdenum Company, Colorado Fuel and Iron Company of Pueblo, and others helped finance the division.

Then a great tragedy occurred. Cummings died in an airplane crash in Utah on December 15, 1942, on his way to give advice to employees of "an essential industry," as Waring phrased it when he read a memorial to him on March 1, 1943. Cummings had assisted in organizing the American Industrial Hygiene Association, serving as president, and published more than thirty scientific articles. The American Industrial Hygiene Association's oldest award is the Donald E. Cummings Memorial Award.

As Cummings's successor, Fred R. Ingram was asked "to acquire field measuring instruments, equip and set up a chemical laboratory and hire personnel. The School of Medicine provided the space," according to Jane McGilvray, a laboratory technician in the division. William McGilvray, her husband—a prisoner of war in Germany—came home and went to work in the division as an industrial hygiene engineer. Franklin Church, an industrial engineer and chemist, joined the staff in November 1943.

A well-equipped chemical laboratory was established early in 1944, and a year later, the biologic and the chemical laboratories merged. Originally housed in the basement of the main hospital building, the division was given space in a new wing built after the war.

In May 1944 the division began a study of exposure to cadmium at the Globeville Plant of American Smelting and Refining. It also conducted contract work for Colorado Fuel and Iron and Climax Molybdenum. Molybdenum is a metallic element used in steel manufacturing, and Climax—located on the Continental Divide—produced a large proportion of the output of the United States. In May 1946 Waring applied for a research grant-in-aid for "investigation of toxicity of various heavy metals (particularly cadmium) and the maximum atmospheric and biologic concentrations which can be withstood without injury to the individual." Ruth Waring Halpenny worked in the laboratory for several months in 1945 and 1946 testing human biological specimens for cadmium and lead. "New equipment was always appearing," she says, "requiring updating of our methods of analysis and resulting in greater accuracy."

Dr. Jonas E. Schreider, who was with the division for nine months until called into military service, describes his work:

> The division . . . was concerned with the problem of silicosis, which was fairly common because many men had mined the 'hard rock' in years past . . . and left many of the miners with silicosis of the lungs that frequently led to tuberculosis. A competent worker had published a paper that stated that aluminum powder when breathed would counteract the silicon. Later another stated that the aluminum would reverse the action of the silicon.

Research was conducted along these lines but failed to show any benefit to breathing aluminum powder.

Dr. George Wright, a physiologist, knew Waring through his work as head of the pulmonary function laboratory of the Edward L. Trudeau Foundation at Saranac Lake; he later became a professor in the Department of Medicine at Case-Western Reserve. Wright's laboratory also conducted aluminum dust experiments: "The idea," he said, "was to prevent, not treat, silicosis. In both animal and human exposures, it failed. . . . Dr. Waring developed interest in occupational and infectious lung diseases in the people he'd trained. Through my periodic contacts with him at Saranac Lake, he influenced me. He always knew where knowledge needed to be developed; he knew what we don't know. [He was] active in getting people to develop new information, stimulated others."

By 1945, medical students at the University of Colorado spent one hour per week throughout the junior year learning the basic principles of industrial hygiene. An elective course was offered seniors that included additional field and laboratory work and research opportunities. In the late 1940s, when the medical school was making major curriculum revisions, a block of time was given to industrial medicine by Dr. Frank Princi, who had joined the division, later becoming director. After Waring asked for support, a grant of $5,000 was approved by the regents of the University of Colorado, and in 1947 the Rockefeller Foundation gave $4,000 for research and equipment. All the while the Warings continued their personal support.

The division's activities grew to include contracts with the Atomic Energy Commission, the Denver Police Department (toxicological tests), the American Cancer Society, and more. By 1945 the division had worked for mines, steel works, smelters, battery plants, creameries, lead works, foundries, structural steel works, and potteries. Besides investigating working conditions in various industries, the division also supervised the establishment of industrial hygiene departments within the plants of several of its clients. Among the division's long-range contributions was its work leading to legislation on the amount of toxins in the air, recalls Jane McGilvray, who says her husband testified several times before legislative committees.

In the mid-1950s, the division merged with the Division of Preventive Medicine, taking that name. Although Waring was extremely interested in preventive medicine, his reaction to seeing the division combined with another is not known. The merger may have resulted from a need to pare costs: By combining the two divisions, the cost of each was reduced. Furthermore, mining became less important, and silicosis studies became the main thrust of the division.

For whatever reasons, and there no doubt were many, the industrial medicine division met its demise when much more knowledge still was needed. The environmental movement had yet to appear; Rachel Carson's *Silent Spring* had not yet been written; the Environmental Protection Agency did not exist. Ahead of his time in recognizing the influence of industrial medicine upon health and the environment, Waring showed courage, motivation, and perseverance in undertaking his pioneering work in the field.

9 *Wartime*

WITH THE OUTBREAK of war in Europe in September 1939, it seemed only a matter of time before the United States would be drawn into the conflict. A shift took place in U.S. neutrality in September 1940 when President Franklin D. Roosevelt transferred fifty destroyers to Great Britain in exchange for naval bases on the Atlantic Coast and elsewhere. It seems probable that James Waring approved of the lend-lease program, for the following year he telegraphed one Colorado senator: "It seems inevitable that we will get into this war. I am greatly disturbed at slowness with which United States is getting ready. I am also alarmed at mounting spiral of prices and wages. Please support Gore price-fixing bill. Authorize arming merchant ships and navy to escort American ships into belligerent ports as may be necessary to give effective aid to Britain."

After the United States entered the war, the ranks of the medical school's faculty rapidly became depleted; eventually about half joined the armed forces. On January 5, 1942, the School of Medicine adopted the accelerated plan, giving the four-year medical course in three calendar years by eliminating summer vacation. Despite a shortage of teachers, high standards were maintained. Under the accelerated plan, the school turned out forty or more new doctors every nine months for the army and navy. Rosters of the Department of Medicine for 1942–1943 show that Waring was listed for service on all the wards for the entire year. In a letter of December 1943, he told of the shortage of doctors to help on the wards and teach students: "We used to have five men, now only one, and that one is going to quit." There were fewer interns and residents as well.

Besides his usual work at the medical school and in private consultations, in 1941 Waring became president of the American Clinical and Climatological Association. At some point he was asked to serve as civilian consultant to the surgeon general, visiting military hospitals that dealt with tuberculosis patients. He went to the Pacific Coast to investigate the handling of cases returning from the Pacific Theater, and in the El Paso area he made ward rounds and gave clinics, as well as inspecting prisoner of war camps. A clipping from a Savannah paper—

no name or date—tells that Waring served on the Subcommittee on Tuberculosis of the Committee on Medicine of the National Research Council in Washington and was studying unidentified medical problems arising out of the Selective Service, especially those concerning tuberculosis. In a letter to a colleague, he later observed, "Largely because of the insistence of this committee, x-ray photographs were made of all men entering military service."

Other wartime assignments came to him. In 1943 he was one of three doctors attending a three-day course in "Chemical Warfare Medicine" in Chicago (his daughter Anne recalls that the concept of chemical warfare upset him immensely), and on December 15, 1943, he visited a prisoner of war camp in Lordsburg, New Mexico.

The West was also the site of internment camps for Japanese Americans. Dr. Shimpei Sakaguchi, whose father bought a farm in Brighton, Colorado, grew up in nearby Henderson. When Sakaguchi, a pediatric surgeon, was a senior in the University of Colorado School of Medicine, Waring paid him to help with medical abstracts. Sakaguchi recalled that he was paid "something like 30 cents an hour" by the National Youth Administration. "I needed the money," he said. "Dr. Waring would assign me things to read and abstract for him. I got paid for learning." Sakaguchi applied various places for a rotating internship but was turned down. A vacancy was created when a classmate was offered another option, at which point Drs. Waring and Mugrage arranged for Sakaguchi to intern at Colorado General Hospital. "Dr. Waring was such a gentle man; I think he liked everybody," Sakaguchi remembered. "At rounds he treated everyone so graciously. . . . I'm just grateful for what he did for me; he supported me all the way."

Waring's responsibilities at the medical school continued unabated. In 1941 he served on ten of fourteen committees and subcommittees and chaired two—more than any other faculty member. He reduced the number by one in 1943, but in 1944 he was again on ten committees and chairman of two. When he received a communication from Dr. Vannevar Bush, the head of the U.S. Office of Scientific Research and Development, asking him to contribute to a report on the future of medical research in the United States, he characteristically said he would. He went to the dean, faculty and regents and solicited their thoughts and convictions. Few who took part in the survey envisioned that an entirely new era was coming, an era in which government money for medical research was so abundant some would call it "The Golden Age of Medicine."

Government money was anything but abundant during the war. As part of a belt-tightening measure because of a shortfall in the state legislature's appropriation for Colorado General Hospital for 1941-1943, it was decided that Ward A—exclusively for tuberculosis patients—would be closed. Later, in 1944, Waring reported that $10,000 had been made available to the School of Medicine for the study of tuberculosis, the study to be directed by himself, and he raised the possibility of reopening Ward A for postgraduate instruction.

Through the years, Waring remained concerned about the need for curriculum change. He wanted less didactic teaching and more bedside teaching time; he also wanted a special committee appointed to study how final examinations were being devised and administered. These topics would be addressed in the postwar period; in the meantime, he kept pushing for reform in other areas. In 1941 he pointed out the inadequacy of equipment in Central Supply; in 1942, he called attention to the failure of many of the outpatient departments to keep records of diagnoses made in the wards; in 1944, his was the one dissenting faculty vote when the age limit for patients admitted to pediatric wards in Colorado General Hospital was raised from twelve to sixteen.

ASTONISHING as it may seem today, in the early 1940s Waring still was not receiving a salary, although he had been professor of medicine and head of the department since 1933. The situation at the University of Colorado School of Medicine was no different from that of many such institutions.[27] However, with the advent of World War II, government support of clinical research began to increase, soon overshadowing private philanthropy and encouraging full-time faculty appointments. An article of May 21, 1941, from a Denver newspaper stated that Waring, "heretofore head of the Department of Medicine on a part-time basis, will retire from his private practice next fall to become full-time head of the Department of Medicine." It said that his salary would be $6,000 a year and that he would be permitted to act as a consultant.

The article was premature: Four years later Waring was granted a salary for his full-time teaching and as head of the Department of Medicine. Why the delay? There were various barriers to the granting of the salary, including opposition from members of the clinical faculty, the basic scientists, and Denver physicians not connected with the medical school. A stringent budget and other considerations also played a part.

Waring offered a motion on August 3, 1942, that the Executive Faculty approve consultation work for full-time members of the faculty, "provided such work does not interfere with the duties of these men in their work in the medical school and hospitals." The motion passed. In

1943 the Public Policy Committee of the Colorado Medical Society recommended that salaries of all full-time heads of departments and their associates at the medical school be raised.

The committee also suggested that full-time faculty be allowed the privilege of consultation, the fees to be collected by the university. In 1944 Dean Rees informed the president of the university, Dr. Robert Stearns, that "Dr. Waring is again becoming somewhat restless on account of our inability to place him on a salary basis. I have explained our budgetary problems and the impossibility of securing funds for this salary." Waring wanted to see a principle upheld. How else would his successor and other faculty members be assured of receiving what they had been told they would? How could well-qualified people be recruited so that the department would flourish?

Next, the Board of Regents ruled that physicians on the medical school faculty who did outside consultation work must give their fees to the school. Waring opposed this ruling, which, he wrote Dean Rees, was "to appease some of our unappeasable colleagues downtown." He pointed out that doctor-teachers needed to supplement their small salaries. A committee of basic science professors came back with a letter to the dean protesting inequities proposed in salaries between the departments. Waring served on a committee formed to iron out differences. Through a conciliatory recommendation, the committee patched together an agreement that would lead to a resolution of the festering problem of faculty pay. The regents finally approved the concept of consultation, with the understanding that full-time professors would offer their expertise only on the invitation of a private doctor. But in 1945, concerned about the number of consultantships opening with the Veterans Administration, Public Health Service and other government services, the regents approved a resolution of the Executive Faculty limiting consultantships to one-sixth of a faculty member's time, one day per week. (These arrangements held until the 1960s and the start of the Faculty Practice Fund.)[28]

Robert L. Stearns, LL.D., who became president of the University of Colorado in 1939 following his term as dean of the School of Law, wrote Waring, his friend of over thirty years: "It is understood that you will retire from active practice as soon as you can do so without prejudice to the interests of your patients and that during the period of your professorship you will have consultation privileges on the same basis as other full-time members of the staff, namely at such times and places as will not interfere with your duties and obligations to the University."

Waring's acceptance letter said that he had been gradually withdrawing from active practice for several years and had been turning work over to his associates, Drs. Robert S. and William A. Liggett: "This past year I have averaged only two visits weekly to my office. Before I became Professor of Medicine, I averaged eleven visits regularly to my office each week. By 'visits' I mean morning or afternoon sessions . . . . My heart is in the University and its School of Medicine. Rest assured that it will be my primary interest at all times."

On May 25, 1945, Dean Rees died. He had taken on the deanship in 1927 and assumed additional duties as superintendent of hospitals, a long tenure during difficult years. Ward Darley, who was full time in the Department of Medicine, in July 1945 was appointed acting dean of the School of Medicine, marking the beginning of what came to be known as "the Darley years."

Summing up the war years, in a letter written in March 1945, a few months before the war's end, Waring wrote to a faculty member serving in the Army that teaching had not deteriorated: "Full time [faculty], volunteer, elderly, 4F have carried on." A card he had filled out for the Civilian Defense Auxiliary provided a rare glimpse into his vital statistics—Age: 59; Height: 5'11"; Hair: ?; Eyes: brown; Color: W.

And he couldn't resist writing "F" for Sex.

FAMILY TIES remained important to James Waring. After his mother died, he visited Savannah at least once each year to see Antonio and his family and Aunt Minna. Antonio called him "son" in some of his letters, his old name within the family. Their cousin, Houstoun Waring, says, "Jim taught me the value of family ties." In the meantime, Waring's own daughters were growing up. With her graduation from Mount Vernon Seminary impending, Ruth looked at various eastern women's colleges but was unhappy with all of them for one reason or another. Then she saw pictures of Wellesley and decided to go there, particularly because it had a good chemistry department. Anne followed her there a year later, majoring in sociology. Whenever he was in the East, their father tried to get together with them. Sometimes he dropped them whimsical notes, such as this one to Anne, which began with a limerick he cut from a magazine and pasted on the letter:

> A girl attending Bryn Mawr
> Committed a dreadful faux pas.
> She loosened a stay
> In her décolleté
> Exposing her je-ne-sais-quoi.

> Dearest Anne, All goes well with us and we hope with you. You have our permission to go on the ski trip. I hope you have a grand time and do not rip your "décolleté" and expose your "je-ne-sais-quoi!" Also, take care of yourself and don't break any bones.

The Farm was closer than Hilltop, and the latter was used less and less. With the advent of war and gas rationing, and with Waring's added responsibilities, there were many reasons not to travel so far, and Hilltop was sold. One of the advantages of having The Farm was that the farmers who looked after the place—a succession of three men over a period of years—grew fresh vegetables, fruits, and flowers. Joe Lind, one of the farmers who ran The Farm, made some improvements, adding a grand root cellar and smoke house. Anne learned skeet and trap shooting with her father on The Farm with the help of Lind, who worked a rather primitive contraption that threw the clay pigeons. Waring, having learned how to raise poultry when he was convalescing in Colorado Springs, enjoyed selecting and ordering the birds raised at The Farm. In 1941, for instance, he ordered broad-breasted turkeys and Cornish chickens, writing to three different dealers.

During the war, Ruth had a "victory garden" with neighbors, which she tended with help. She worked hard for the Red Cross, serving as chapter vice chairman and Washington representative for the American Red Cross. Waring wrote her in January 1943 from a subzero Minneapolis that he hoped she was "strutting your uniform with all your brass and badges." When Ruth was away and he was at home, he missed her as much as ever. Waring could never really be happy when she was gone, although he tried to make light of it. May 1944: "The house seems very quiet without you. Didn't realize you made such a noise around the place."

He continued on his strenuous trips, despite admitting that he was exhausted. The girls were now grown up, but his deep attachment to his family never lessened. Gradually, during the 1940s, when he was traveling to meetings or away at a favorite fishing spot, telephone calls began to replace letters, but a few of the latter survive. In a letter to his wife from Boston, on a day when he had gone past Wellesley, he wrote, "My heart turned over—as it always does at visions real or imaginary of them and you." His notes home usually addressed issues of a personal nature, family affairs, or comments on his trip, but on June 7, 1944, he wrote: "D-Day seems to be going well" the day after the allied assault had begun on the beaches of France. Sometimes he lapsed into his own special lingo: "A good knop last knight and pheeling phitt."

IN THE YEAR following her graduation in 1944 Ruth worked in an industrial laboratory in Virginia, which she now admits was not a good choice. The plant made radar housings of plastic, impregnated fiberglass, and it was her job to test the resins. Although the job did not suit her—"Lab work was too routine; I like variety"—her stay in Marion, not far from Roanoke, was memorable for reasons of the heart.

She started going to services at the Episcopal church in Marion during Lent, and there she met a conscientious objector working in the mental hospital in the town. Would she marry him? A few weeks later she brought her suitor to Denver for a visit. Her parents thought the union unsuitable, and she was talked out of any thought of marrying. (Among Waring's papers is a pamphlet issued by the Society of Friends on "Tolerance," relevant to conscientious objectors, dating from about this time.) The young man later attended a theological seminary and became a minister; Ruth quit her job, returned to Denver, and took nurse's-aid training through the Red Cross at St. Joseph Hospital. Whatever her thoughts may have been about her parents' intrusion into her matrimonial plans, she kept them to herself.

A frequent visitor to The Farm in the 1940s was Dr. Harriot Hunter (later Mrs. Robert Jardine), originally from Savannah. A psychiatrist and graduate of Johns Hopkins School of Medicine, she arrived in Denver during the war and attended Thanksgiving dinner at the Warings' in 1942 along with another guest, music teacher and conductor Antonia Brico. Jardine recalls Waring as "a gentleman par excellence."

During the next three years, she says, "I was busy with a psychiatry residency. Waring would meet me in the hall [at Colorado General Hospital] or at a lecture, chat, invite me out to The Farm. I met his daughters and became very friendly with Anne, a lifelong friendship."[29]

JUNE 1945 was a busy time for Waring. He went to San Francisco to examine for the American Board of Internal Medicine and to receive an award, the Gold-Headed Cane. It would be hard to say which of his many honors meant the most to him, but from the point of view of his interest in medical history, this award was unique.

Dr. William J. Kerr, professor of medicine at the University of California, was largely responsible for bringing the Gold-Headed Cane to the United States. After working in Britain for some time and receiving the cane himself, Kerr in 1939 started a new series of awards for senior medical students at the University of California "based upon the student's interest in the welfare of his patients during his entire clinical experience." Later the award was given to notable physicians in other parts of the country. Drs. Kerr and Waring met at one of the Association of American Physicians meetings, and, in a letter to Paul Anderson, Kerr stated that he "was immediately struck by his charm and intellect. As time passed we became very warm friends."

In the ceremony, held June 23, 1945, Kerr addressed Waring as one of his "idols" in the profession of medicine because of his "scholarly ability and his interest in the welfare of the profession and the students." Waring spoke, characteristically, on "The Life and Work of Laënnec."

Kerr's dedication of the cane to Waring:

> If this Gold-Headed Cane could speak, it would say:
> "I am the reincarnation of the old Gold-Headed Cane.
> "My golden head has been fashioned from the treasure of the hills of California, and my shaft from an ancient yew growing beside a rushing mountain stream.
> "I have watched your career through many decades and marked your contributions to the science and the art of medicine.
> "I have noted with satisfaction your spirit of cooperation with your colleagues and your inspiration to students.
> "I have been aware of your devotion as a physician to the welfare of your patients.
> "I have read the record of the many, well-deserved honors which have been bestowed upon you.
> "I am now intrusted to your keeping in the hope that if some day you find another who exemplifies to a high degree the qualities of the true physician, you will pass me on so that I may be a continuing symbol of all that is good in American medicine."[30]

Four years after he received the cane, Waring established a similar award at the University of Colorado School of Medicine. Each year since, a "cane award" has been presented to the senior medical student who best displays those stellar qualities—clinical ability and devotion to patients—that the cane has represented for the past three hundred years. The honoree receives not a cane but a copy of the seventh edition of *The Gold-Headed Cane,* written in 1827 by a London doctor, William Macmichael. Waring wrote a foreword for the seventh edition (1953), which begins: "'Tradition wears a snowy beard.' America is young, romantic, altruistic, impulsive, materialistic at times, always independent and freedom-loving. . . . The concept of the physician as a man of scholarly attainments as well as professional skills, exemplified in the lives and teachings of the four great Hopkins' doctors, Osler, Welch, Halsted, and Kelly, has not been lost with their passing. You will find it alive not only in Baltimore, Philadelphia and Boston, but in American medical centers far removed from the Atlantic Coast." He concluded: "Tradition . . . will die with neglect and flourish with recognition. Those who cherish tradition will, in scriptural phrase, hold up Dr. Kerr's hands."

The history of the cane was known to Waring before he was made a caneholder, for even before 1945 he had adopted as his bookplate the Chelsea Physic Garden, associated with the original holders of the cane. Allen True executed the design, which features a seventeenth-century figure standing at the gateway to the garden, leaning upon a cane. The five holders of the original cane are named.[31] Other clues can be found to Waring's long-held interest in the cane, for as far back as 1925 he wrote to Ruth from New York City about a bookseller who "wanted $25 for a third edition 1884 of the Gold-Headed Cane and $75 for a second edition which I bought in beautiful condition for $8."

Always delighted to find a family connection, he wrote in a letter to Aunt Minna in 1952: "One of the holders of the Gold-Headed Cane was a very famous and a very fine man by the name of Richard Mead. His second wife was named Anne Alston. [James Waring's maternal grandmother was an Alston]. She was the daughter of Sir Roland Alston." There was a Savannah connection, too: The eighteenth-century Trustees' Garden in Savannah (so-named for James Oglethorpe and his associates, or trustees, who had established the colony of Georgia) was influenced by the Apothecaries' Garden, or Chelsea Physic Garden.

James Waring wrote in his foreword to *The Gold-Headed Cane* that the story of the cane brings "the art of medicine more forcibly to the attention of students, faculty, and to all those concerned with the care of patients. . . . The cane is rescued from obscurity to walk again, a symbol, the outward and visible sign of the attributes of mind and heart of the true physician."

This is what has happened, as periodically the cane was passed on to outstanding practitioners of internal medicine. The determination of the next recipient is made by the present holder. Included among those so honored were Drs. John Ryan (to whom Waring passed the cane), Constantine Kemper, Robert Liggett, Karl Arndt, Gordon Meiklejohn, S. Gilbert Blount, and Stuart Schneck. The most recent recipient of the cane, Dr. William Robinson, an oncologist, is the first recipient to have received the award as a student. The wheel—in this case, the cane—has come full circle.

Part Five | *A Time of Change*

10 | *Postwar Developments*

SHORTHANDED for a long time, the Department of Medicine saw its ranks replenished at war's end. Robert Liggett, a major in the Army Medical Corps, was appointed full-time associate professor of medicine effective September 1, 1946. Waring had a close relationship with his former student and partner, who bought several acres at The Farm and had a house built there.

Dr. Hope Lowry, a graduate of Johns Hopkins, became the fourth full-time member of the department. Along with Dr. Leighton Anderson, a general internist, and Dr. John W. Berry, director of the Outpatient Department, she took her turn visiting on the tuberculosis ward and in the general medical wards. Dr. Abe Ravin also was active in teaching, as was Dr. William Liggett—Robert's brother—who was appointed instructor. The medical school continued to rely upon the help of volunteer faculty.

In 1947 Ward Darley became vice president of the University of Colorado and dean of the medical center. In 1949 the positions were divided, and Darley was made vice president of the university and director of the medical center; Dr. Robert C. Lewis became dean.

Lowry's appointment was considered something of a milestone in 1946, a time when few women in this country were full-time faculty members. She says that in general Waring was opposed to women in medicine, "but he always qualified the statement by saying, 'Hope, I don't mean you!'" Harriot Hunter Jardine disagrees with Lowry's view that he had any bias. Whatever his thoughts on the subject, the enrollment of women in the School of Medicine was gradually increasing. By January 1948, of 239 medical students, 24 were women.

Lowry is candid: "Dr. Waring was not universally loved." She saw him day in and day out and was aware of run-ins he had had with other departments or with those who were not doing their jobs according to his standards. She tells of how he took a careful history, did a meticulous physical exam, and used humor to interest and wake up the students—such as his advice about a rectal exam: "If you don't put your finger in it, you put your foot in it." Lowry says he was not "a benevolent Santa Claus. He was a spicier man." What he was: "A great physician, a bedside physician. . . . He was a marvelous clinician, marvelous diagnostician. [Such doctors] don't exist today."

Dr. Henry Swan II (no relation to Will Howard Swan, James Waring's doctor in Colorado Springs), appointed assistant professor of surgery, later would become the first full-time professor of surgery at the University of Colorado School of Medicine. Swan recalls that he was a college student when he first met Waring—his father was a friend of Waring. His maternal grandfather was Dr. Charles Denison, who interested Waring, Swan says, because of his work in pulmonary medicine. "Denison made climatic and geographic studies and weather maps. He was an inventor, too; he invented a device to expand or collapse the lung."

The professor of medicine and the new member of the surgical staff helped bring the two departments closer. Swan states:

> Back in Boston there were the clinical-pathological conferences at Massachusetts General [Hospital], the key element being that all services were there. They'd try to make lessons of the case escape the bounds of specialization. . . . [In Colorado] I helped work out the format with Dr. Waring. Different departments presented one or two cases per week in the Sabin Amphitheater. All students attended in the last two years of school.
>
> We wanted to make the point that the two departments [medicine and surgery], unlike the usual political game, would establish the ideal that internecine warfare wasn't a good idea. Interests of patient came first. Dr. [E. Stewart] Taylor [obstetrics/gynecology] liked the idea. Radiology, pathology, all services were represented, attended by all the house staff.

Swan tells of the small cafeteria for faculty, which seated twenty-five to forty people. "[The small cafeteria] was a good thing because basic science doctors and clinical doctors got together. During the years of development, 1946–1956, the medical school was a reasonably compact group."

Another change in the postwar years was in the increasing availability of federal funds for medical research. On January 22, 1946, President Gustavson wrote Waring:

> The Regents expressed very positive interest in research and hope that the university will grow in this particular field of activity. They also asked me to tell you that they will be very happy to receive

> federal grants covering the field of medical research. I explained to them that such grants were never given with the demand that people carry out work in a certain way. They seemed anxious to safeguard the liberty of the investigator, and I assured them that his liberty and freedom as an investigator was never involved in research grants.

Two months later Waring reported to the Executive Faculty Committee on the meetings of the Committee on Scientific Research, to be held in Denver in March. The committee as a whole, he said, appeared to favor receiving funds from the federal government for medical research. In light of the present-day dependence on federal grants, this attitude toward government involvement seems somewhat wary.

In September Waring proposed that an isotope committee be appointed to deal with the problems of the purchase and use of radioactive materials for medical research. He chaired a committee appointed in 1946 to address these concerns. In 1947, the Annual Survey of Research in Progress of the Research Committee of the medical center stated:

> It has become increasingly difficult for the Dean and the Committee to keep in accurate touch with the various research projects underway within the Medical Center. . . . The faculty have been very successful in their attempts to bring outside research funds into the institution. The contrast between the financial support available for research before the war and the support it enjoys today is very striking. [In 1948 the School of Medicine received an appropriation of $1,200,000 for cancer research.] The committee is concerned, however, at the possibility that the many plans involving increased teaching and other non-research duties for faculty members may prevent the faculty from accomplishing all they should and can in research.

A priority of the medical school now was revitalization of the curriculum, with all the changes that technology, research, and the new frontiers of medicine were bringing. Darley had addressed the changing needs in a report dated December 4, 1944:

> Prior to World War II the School of Medicine was an undergraduate institution devoted almost solely to training M.D.s. The Medical School would need, after the war, to become a medical center: teaching young men and women to become physicians, training

> interns, nurses and technicians, offering graduate and postgraduate opportunities to general physicians, specialists, and basic scientists, providing the best in medical care to patients in the hospitals and clinics, and performing biological and medical research.

The curriculum would have to be revamped. In 1947 Dean Darley asked Swan to set up committees and subcommittees to plan for the clinical and preclinical years. Waring had strong views on the subject and had been making them known for years. He was not, however, on a major committee, only on the history of medicine subcommittee. One active participant in the curriculum-revamping process says that Waring was overburdened at the time and wanted to get rid of some of his duties, "letting his old friend Bob Liggett take some of them." Liggett was on the Committee for Integration of Clinical Teaching and several subcommittees.

Swan, who came to know Waring as a friend ("One of the earliest things we had in common was fishing"), says of him: "He was a true aristocrat. People wanted to emulate him. [He had] wit, humor, intelligence. He was a leader among men." But he also was "controversial. [He incited] envy. That's inevitable." The surgeon was no stranger to controversy himself. A pioneer in cardiac surgery, using hypothermia in open-heart surgery in the days before the heart-lung machine had been invented, Swan recalled that a lot of negative publicity about his work was carried in the local newspapers: "'Subsidized by state,' they said. Papers were full of it. Jim was supportive of me. He'd call me in consultation for patients on the medical service."

In 1946 the House of Delegates of the Colorado Medical Society passed a resolution that stressed the importance of adequately educating physicians and pledged its "militant support of a legislative program for increased appropriations to the University of Colorado to the end that the University's School of Medicine may obtain that degree of excellence" outlined in the introductory statement.

An added impetus for the society's strong support may have been the health crisis then facing in the state. A poliomyelitis epidemic was threatening the population, taxing the facilities and personnel of medical institutions. In the course of 1946, 303 poliomyelitis patients were admitted to Colorado General Hospital; 900 cases occurred statewide. The facilities at Colorado General were severely strained, with most of the beds filled by polio patients, and with all the tank respirators, or "iron lungs," constantly in use by patients with respiratory muscle paralysis. Many had a combined bulbar-respiratory muscle paralysis.

There were so many respirator patients that Colorado General took the adults, and the children went to Children's Hospital. Denver General Hospital stepped in and took patients who normally would have gone to Colorado General but had to go elsewhere because of a shortage of beds. Teamwork by all was essential.

Dr. Winona Campbell, a volunteer pediatric faculty member, helped care for both children and adults in the hospital.[32] In 1947 Campbell, as the attending physician on the polio service, was working entirely with adults. The adult care was under the supervision of Waring, who would make rounds almost every day. She would go into his office each morning from 11 A.M. to noon. "It was a great privilege to have as close contact as I had with Waring," she says. "After lunch we discussed patients. He was a great clinician, very astute. We all loved him."[33]

On August 12, 1947, the day after James Waring's sixty-fourth birthday, Dean Darley read a letter from Waring stating that he wished to resign as head of the Department of Medicine effective April 1, 1948. He would, however, continue as a full-time professor in the department. Teaching was his special interest and he was not ready to relinquish that role, but he needed relief from administrative responsibilities, greater now than ever before. Some of the coming changes already were apparent–the rise of subspecialties and the growing emphasis on research. Meeting the demands of these new trends required great energy. The dean appointed a special committee to consider Waring's request and the issues he had raised. In the interim, Robert Liggett, assistant dean, was appointed acting head of the department.

Waring's involvement in national organizations had brought credit to the university. From 1938 to 1944 he was a governor of the American College of Physicians; in 1946 he became a life member and first vice-president and in 1948 a master—one of four physicians in the United States and Canada to receive this honor, bestowed upon him at the annual meeting in New York City, "for outstanding teaching service and medical research." He was a pioneer in board certification in the field of internal medicine, recognized as one of the men who instilled the high standards of accreditation in this specialty. In 1946 he wrote Ruth from Buffalo: "Attended a very interesting meeting of the Council of the Trudeau Society at which I had to take a very active part in protesting unwise suggestions to change the methods of certification by the American Board of Internal Medicine."

Now he was trying to cut back: "Told Bill Werrell I was thru with ABIM [American Board of Internal Medicine] this year," he wrote to Ruth from Chicago in 1947. "He looked crushed which was tactful."

The previous year he had been chairman of the organization, of which he had been a founder in 1936. Yet for every responsibility he dropped, he seemed to find another to replace it. In 1948 he gave several lectures in the West—Salt Lake City, Seattle, and Vancouver, British Columbia, giving four papers and conducting a clinic at the latter. In truth, he was cutting back only moderately.

HUMOR was an integral part of Waring's personality, and he became known as a very funny man. Best known, perhaps, was Waring the raconteur. His storytelling ability went back to his upbringing. Houstoun Waring, recalling the embellished tales at 1229 Race Street, says his cousin "turned incidents into yarns." Waring told anecdotes in lectures and conversation not only to entertain but also to instruct, using both ethnic and rural humor deeply rooted in the old South. A favorite was the tale of the country girl at a southern dance who was left without an invitation to dance for a long period of time. When finally asked to dance, she responded, in a strong backwoods accent, "Thankya' very much, sir, I 'most took root!"

The teller of dialect and ethnic jokes, of course, risks being labeled as prejudiced. Some who heard Waring's jokes may have perceived them as insensitive, but most listeners fell under the spell of the storyteller. Part of the magic was his voice, the twinkle in his eyes, or his use of body English—seeing him, for example, flapping his elbow-wings in his best seagull manner, forming a bird's beak by connecting his thumbs, telling a story about a mother seagull flying over a Harvard-Yale rowing meet with her young:

> "What is that?" asked a baby seagull.
> "The Poughkeepsie Regatta."
> "What's that?"
> "A boat race."
> "Who's winning?"
> "I don't know," said the mother seagull, "but I put everything I had on Harvard."

Ruth tells of her father's lightheartedness, labeling some of his tales as being "often ribald, sometimes in mixed company, depending upon the company." Anne tells how her father relished telling jokes using an accent, such as the time when he slipped a worm into a patient's pan, whereupon—as he later told it—a nurse rushed out of the patient's room, calling excitedly, "Dr. Varing! Dr. Varing! The patient has womited a vorm!"

Above all, says Anne, her father liked spontaneous humor. She tells of the time she was traveling with him in the South and they had a long wait for a train. Suddenly he stood up, put down his newspaper and, in the accent of the conductor, shouted that such and such a train was leaving on such and such track—"All a-bawd!"—then sat down and put his head back inside the paper.

Former students also have recollections of their professor's playfulness. Dr. Robert K. Brown, a chest surgeon, tells a story of Waring looking at an x-ray of a well-endowed young woman and pronouncing "TB." The astonished students could see no such indication.

"Two beauts," was the professor's explanation.

Most remembrances, however, are more thoughtful—such as this long, anonymous letter that arrived with Waring's Christmas mail in 1942:

> You are no doubt well aware how highly we respect you . . . Nor do I stand alone in my appreciation of what you have done for us . . . . There isn't a dissenter in the group when anyone speaks highly of "Uncle Jim."
>
> You wonder what has happened to all this respect when we call you "Uncle Jim." To students of the C.U. Medical School the term "Uncle" has a very special connotation. . . . It's a title we use only affectionately when we have a very high degree of respect and love for the recipient. . . .[34]
>
> Your scholarliness in medicine has won you respect but it is your sense of humor, and your ability to appreciate the other fellow's situation that has won for you the undying endearment of the class. . . . A Senior Student.

At some time, perhaps in the late 1930s, Waring had become known as "Gentleman Jim" because of his respect for students and his aversion to embarrassing them. Some, as in the letter above, affectionately called him "Uncle Jim," even "Lord Jim," but it was "Gentleman Jim" by which he was best known. Liggett called Waring "humble, easy for students to talk to," adding: "He didn't in any way hold anyone off. This was why students admired him. They could stop him anywhere and ask him anything, and he always had the time to talk with them. . . . He had a sense of humor which he used to put over important points, which really impressed you and enabled you to remember the point he was trying to put across." Ward Darley cited Waring as "a superb teacher who had much more of an impact on me than any other physician I could name." Dr. Charles Freed, class of 1933, who had a rotating internship under Waring, recalled: "I have specialized in neurology and neurosurgery and have met many great physicians, surgeons, and scholars. I don't think any of them were better teachers or physicians than Dr. Waring."

Dr. Lula Lubchenco, a distinguished neonatologist and one of four women out of forty-nine students in the class of 1939, states, "We all thought of him as the professor. He was revered." She describes an episode in which he helped her answer questions in cardiology: "During one of our class lectures I was asked to come down in front of the class and read an EKG [electrocardiogram]. The EKG contained many extra systoles, or premature beats. When a premature beat occurs there is a pause until the next beat before the normal rhythm resumes. I couldn't remember what a pause in the rhythm was called. He was kind; he tried to give me hints: 'You have a boyfriend and you had a date but he couldn't come, so he sent a dozen roses.'" Then it came to her: "Compensatory!"

Dr. Michael Lubchenco, a brother of Lula Lubchenco and a general surgeon until arthritis forced him to give up his practice, served twenty years as director of medical education at Presbyterian Hospital in Denver. He remembered: "We had a wartime shortage of faculty; many of the clinical professors were so busy they didn't show up for lectures. [Dr. Waring would] take us to National Jewish Hospital, not only for sessions on tuberculosis but for physical diagnosis. It was a marvelous place to go and learn auscultation, for example; he'd love to pick up physical findings and demonstrate them to us."

Lubchenco recalled the time that Waring had a private patient referred and "asked me to 'get the history and do the physical.' I rejoined him for rounds. There was not much in the way of physical findings, but the X ray showed a mass. 'You do as I say and not as I do,' Waring said, because he'd missed the mass, too. He had a twinkle that was devilish. . . . You would hate to let him down and would make sure the next time you wouldn't miss something."

Dr. John Durrance, class of 1943 in the wartime accelerated program, transferred from Dartmouth Medical School, which then had only a two-year program. Mountaineer and ski champion, he became head of respiratory diseases at the Denver Veterans Administration Hospital and acquired a reputation for being a very astute chest physician. "As a [medical] student," he says, "I achieved the rare accomplishment of sleeping with my eyes open. During one class on diabetes Dr. Waring caught me, brain disengaged. I didn't know the question, so we fenced. He wouldn't let me off the hook the rest of the session. We were like two lawyers. He never referred to that incident again."

When he was chief resident, Durrance received a call from Waring asking him to examine a patient and feel his spleen. "I thought, 'What a request!'—I was very busy, so made the examination fast and reported that I had felt 'just the tip' of it." Waring asked, "Did you look at his belly?" Told that he had, Waring then asked, "Did you see the scar?" Unbeknownst to Durrance, the patient had recently undergone a splenectomy (removal of the spleen). "He let me remember that afterwards!" For months thereafter, when Waring would encounter a palpable spleen he would call for Jack Durrance, "a man with a fine touch for a very hard-to-feel spleen." Durrance enjoyed it as much as anyone.

Alfred Crowle, Ph.D., tells of Waring's direct ways with students: "He would criticize a student, yet the student would not get angry." Crowle observed a student making a lecture presentation and heard Waring tell him, "'You should not be addressing your um-bil-*i*-cus when you are talking to an audience,'" purposely mispronouncing the word.

Says Dr. Robert Jardine, a general practitioner-geriatrician (and husband of Dr. Harriot Hunter):

> He [Waring] was an excellent instructor; I had him during my junior year as clinical instructor in medicine. Primarily he taught us respiratory diagnosis; he would teach us how to examine a respiratory patient. . . . I saw him examining patients at Denver General; he treated all with a great deal of dignity. I also had the experience of seeing his private patients in consultation.
>
> I was particularly impressed when he'd bring a chest X ray in, then ask a student to discuss it; his ability to pick up subtle changes. After Waring's death I remember having a patient who had a respiratory problem. I looked over the X ray and pointed out insignificant looking changes. "Dr. Waring has been teaching you," said the staff physician in radiology, Bertram Pear. "His students always know so much."

As a teaching tool, Waring often used catchy phrases. He described what could be seen in the x-ray of residual cavities, which could be rendered noninfectious and which he insisted not be removed, as "last year's bird's nests." It was a phrase repeated by a generation of chest physicians.

"The thing everyone looked forward to was grand rounds," said Dr. J. Philip Clarke, an internist and a founder of the Denver Clinic. He spoke of Waring's performance at grand rounds "with live patients, unlike clinical-pathological conferences, which were autopsies with debates between clinicians and pathologists." In his capacity as governor for the Colorado Chapter of the American College of Physicians, Clarke wrote an appreciation of Waring's grand rounds that appeared in *History of the Department of Medicine, 1933–1985.*

> I shall never forget one such performance during my senior year (1945). A young woman with a long progressive illness had died. She had remained a diagnostic dilemma until her death. Dr. Waring analyzed the clinical course, laboratory and radiographic findings, and finally after twenty minutes of discourse came to the magnificent conclusive statement: "This young lady died of Systemic Lupus Erythematosus and Dr. Black (the pathologist) will show us Libman-Sacks lesions in her heart!" Spontaneous cheering and applause ensued and 'Doctor Jim' was proven correct. Now at this time, according to the then current Cecil, only twenty-three cases of Systemic Lupus had been reported—an exceedingly rare disease.
>
> In 1952, Dr. Waring had stepped aside as Department Chairman. But I continued to benefit from his wisdom and advice. One day when I returned from the Denver General Hospital, he asked how things were going. I gave him a two-minute capsule summary of a perplexing case we had seen on the ward that morning. His eyes twinkled as he said, "Don't forget Nocordia!" And Nocordiosis it proved to be—a patient who subsequently was cured relatively easily with a sulfonamide drug. But I also learned about fly fishing, dry-land farming, myotonic disease in goats, pride in his Mastership in the American College of Physicians, and various and sundry bits of knowledge. . . . He had his "warts," as all of us do. At times he could be petulant, jealous and intolerant of the beliefs of others. But for many graduates of the University of Colorado School of Medicine of his era, Dr. Jim Waring served as a major role model, first in attracting us into Internal Medicine as a career, and secondly in stimulating us to emulate so many of the attributes which he, as "the compleat physician," embodied.

Although an expert in respiratory disease, Waring was renowned for his breadth of knowledge, with general expertise in cardiovascular, infectious and metabolic diseases, endocrinology, respiratory physiology, gastroenterology, and psychosomatic physiology. Dr. Robert Weiner, class of 1952, was impressed by the fact that Waring spoke without benefit of notes. "He called himself an 'Old Lunger,'" Weiner recalled.

A student in the postwar period told of the time a visiting professor, who was applying for the position of professor of medicine, was giving a lecture in the amphitheater. When he had finished speaking, the head of the selection committee turned to Waring and asked for comments. As the students and house staff looked at him expectantly, Waring made his way to the podium. His gracious words made an impression on Dr. Walter Huttner: "When the nightingale sings, all the other birds in the forest are still." Then he left the podium and took his seat.

Milton Rees, M.D., class of 1939, recalled Waring's response when a faculty committee decided to discharge a competent but not brilliant student from the Ozark Mountains on the grounds of his "atrocious" backwoods habits, manners, and vocabulary. He paraphrased Waring: "'Do you gentlemen know that this boy's grandmother sits on her porch rocking back and forth and smoking a corn cob pipe and is not able to read or write? As long as I am chief of the medical service and this boy has made such progress . . . I will not permit him to be expelled from this institution unless you expel me first.'"

In a 1949 talk to members of Alpha Omega Alpha, honorary medical society at the University of Utah School of Medicine, Waring reminded them: "The letters AOA stand for the Greek words meaning: 'To be worthy to serve the suffering.'" He asked, "What makes a man worthy to serve the suffering?"

> Scholarship is not enough. Book learning, clinical experience, industry, integrity, certain natural skills are all essential to success, but all these things are cold compared to the heart-warming spirit of compassion. The ability and the never-failing willingness to sit down unhurriedly with the patient and explain to him the nature of his illness and what he must do to be well, are often God given qualities. . . . Some, alas, lack it, even scorn it in others! . . .
>
> I sometimes think that every doctor, every medical student should have early in his career a serious illness, one requiring perhaps only brief hospitalization, but an illness that threatened extended interruption of work, if not life itself—this illness to be part of his medical education.

On more than one occasion Waring was quoted to this effect: "It has been my good fortune to serve three separate and extended hitches as a bed patient, the time so spent numbering in all about nine years." Good fortune? He meant it. Nine years may sound like hyperbole, but it adds up, counting all the years he went to his bed to rest during the day and the specific extended medical crises of 1907–1910, 1919, and 1931–1932.

His patients felt his concern. In a February 1932 letter to Ruth, he said: "From the first I have anticipated disaster with Charlie. . . . Nothing I did for him seemed to do him much good and at the end I became convinced that the new serum upon which I leaned heavily for help failed me and caused bad reactions. My spirit has been terrifically low about it all but I did my very best and [a] man can do no more." But a well-to-do neighbor was infuriated when, after having a physical examination and being found in good health, he was charged twenty-five dollars. The neighbor wanted to have no charge for the examination or else to have the charge reduced. Yet for many of limited means, he charged nothing at all or reduced his fee to five dollars.

Polly Riedeburg Plesset stated: "Dr. Waring really cared . . . [and] didn't give up easily. Didn't suffer fools gladly." She missed most of grade school because of whooping cough, pneumonia, and other illnesses but made up much of the work. She had to wear "great big jackets of mustard plaster" prescribed by her beloved Waring. After an operation for appendicitis, she developed a stitch abscess and was very ill. Waring came to see her every day; only later did she find out that his mother had died about that time.

Virginia Shafroth Newton recalls that when she and her sister Ellen went in for their check-ups, Waring, knowing of Ellen's special athletic talent, would ask her to walk on her hands down the hall!

James Waring's concern would turn to anger when he believed the patient was receiving poor care. Dr. Milton Rees, in correspondence with Paul Anderson in the early 1960s, recalled, "A colored gentleman, with a very unappealing odor due to inadequate hygiene, had been relegated by the students and house staff to a back corner, and somewhat forgotten. When Waring discovered this man and heard that all the attention the patient had received consisted of a 'little piece of glass to suck' [a thermometer], his exasperation and indignation were great."

Other patients were also willing to share their thoughts about the doctor. Kenneth Caughey contracted tuberculosis in 1945 while serving in the Marine Corps in China. Saved by streptomycin, he became sick a second time, and again recovered. In 1953, soon after his marriage, he had another relapse. He went to see Waring and was immediately struck by his concern, compassion, and kindness. Caughey tells about meeting Waring in his office at the medical school. "It was hard to believe such a prominent person would be in such a plain little office. I could tell he had an immediate feeling for what I was going through. . . . It was his manner, which was gentle, but at the same time realistic. Here was a man who had an influence on the rest of my life because of how he approached me and my problem: 'Let's get on with it and get this thing whipped. Then you can go on with your life.'"

He was put to bed at the Denver Veterans Administration Hospital for four months, at first with total bedrest, then gradual activity. Caughey states:

> I went into the TB ward. Dr. Waring came over, I can't tell you how frequently. It always made me feel good just to have him walk through the room. He always had a nice smile. I enjoy fishing, and as you know that was one of his great loves, so we would talk and talk and talk about fishing experiences. . . . I not only became a friend of Dr. Waring, but I learned to love the man. . . . He was compassionate and understanding and he was a super physician, and I knew that the treatment I was receiving was what I should be receiving.

Later on, for many years Caughey—a son-in-law of Robert Stearns—served on the board of the Webb-Waring Lung Institute, no doubt a way of saying thank you to the man who "instilled hope." His wife Judith later wrote of the period in which Ken fell to Waring's care: "We will always be grateful for the wisdom and the gentleness and the humor that helped Ken—and me."

Robert Stearns, also one Waring's patients, wrote a letter in October 1943 extolling the care he had received: "Please be assured that my recovery was due entirely to the skill of that distinguished faculty—without the aid of Waring and Dr. E. A. Schmidt, I am certain that I would have succumbed."

Dr. George Curfman, Jr., a Denver internist, told of an incident illustrating Waring's "Gentleman Jim" way with patients. Curfman came to Denver in 1947 and says he did not see much of Waring until one day when he had a patient with a complicated illness at St. Joseph Hospital. He had trouble making a diagnosis so he called Waring. When Waring arrived, Curfman introduced him to the patient—they already had gone over the case together—and Waring sat at the bedside and asked questions in a "kind, considerate way." "Now Dr. Curfman and I will go out and review your case and I'll offer my opinion," Waring told the patient.

"Dr. Curfman will be happy to review our findings and recommendations with you. It's been a pleasure to see you and talk to you." Forty or so years after this encounter Curfman clearly recalls the conversation. "He was very humble about the whole thing."

The alleviation of mental as well as physical distress is often the task of the doctor. A patient wrote to Waring, "I have been made to see what a thoughtless, selfish, self-centered, undeveloped person I really am. . . . There is already a change going on inside of me. My husband and son deserved a better deal. . . . If only I had better medical help long ago this situation would never have existed. I have never been a person to tell my troubles to someone . . . Why is it that whenever I feel the need for real help you are the one person that comes to my mind. You have given me so many chances and I failed you in all of them. I know this time I will not."

Waring replied: "I was greatly relieved to see how well you looked and how steady you seemed. The thing to do now is to turn your face towards the days ahead and not to spend any time on past troubles and mistakes, if any. I think you are a very fine young woman and I feel very sure that the future holds much happiness and good health for you. Keep busy at outside interests which will help to protect you against becoming introspective. When you feel like it, come to see me."

He did not charge those who could not pay, but included among his patients were many prominent people, such as members of the Phipps family, U.S. Senator Ed Johnson, the Gurtler family (which owned Elitch Gardens, a Denver amusement park), and architect and developer Temple Buell, to name a few. Most patients, of course, were not well-known people. Anne recalls seeing her father cry at the death of a young patient at the medical school.

One of Waring's longtime patient relationships is well documented. Mark H. Harrington spoke at the Waring symposium in 1963, telling of his marriage as a young law student to his wife Lucile in 1932 and his discovery six months later that she had tuberculosis. After a year at the University of Michigan hospital, her condition deteriorated, and she was close to death. A young doctor on the hospital staff from Colorado told him that if it were his wife he would take her to Colorado, for there they would be "close to a man named Waring." Harrington wrote Waring requesting that he care for Lucile and received a letter saying that he would do so. Harrington stated:

> I started for the West (by this time I was down to twenty dollars), bumming my way from Ann Arbor, Michigan, to Denver. When I

> arrived I was just about a pauper, but I managed to get a little work through a friend, and I sent for my wife. On a Sunday morning we lifted her out of the train on a stretcher and took her to a hotel. Dr. Waring came down to the hotel and examined her . . . and finally he said to her, "Lucile, I will see you through." . . . We went to Boulder, where I joined the law school faculty. Dr. Waring used to travel up to Boulder on the old road (about thirty-six miles each way) and then he would send me a bill for five dollars for the consultation. He knew that I had a certain amount of pride and self-respect, and he was going to help me preserve it, and so he sent me a bill for his services. One time on one of these seventy-two-mile round trips he had arranged a conference with a number of doctors in Boulder. They came and examined Lucile, and after the conference was over, one of these doctors said, "This girl will die any hour. She will have the last convulsive closing of the trachea or of the main bronchial tubes and die of suffocation." And I shall never forget what Dr. Waring replied: "While there is life, there is hope," and he would not give her up. . . . He never gave up hope for his patients.

Harrington took a job in Denver so that they would be closer to Waring. He continued:

> On the days that he had visited (and before she told me that he had been there), I could tell the difference in her. She was happy, she was smiling, and she had hope and courage again. And finally, after this long period of time, Lucile regained her health. . . . Dr. Waring had a kind of medicine which was the kind Lucile needed to save her life. That medicine was that he shared his heart with her, and she knew it.

The former patient, Lucile Harrington, recalled:

> My tuberculosis was so far advanced in November of 1933 that Dr. Barnwell of the University of Michigan Hospital felt that the chance of my recovery in going to Colorado was like "finding a needle in a haystack." Dr. Waring told us the story of the young intern who told him that "the bedside manner" was obsolete. The doctor wondered what had taken its place. We didn't think of him as a famous physician because he had the true bedside manner of interest, kindness, and hope. I remember another story he told of a well

> known physician [Dr. Osler] making rounds in a hospital with a group of young doctors. They told him that everything had been done for the patient, but he could not live. He answered, "And what have you left for the Lord to do?"

Although James Waring was not considered by some to be a religious person, others knew he was. Mark Harrington stated: "Dr. Waring was a religious man. I don't mean that he paraded his religion, but he practiced his religion, and he knew a great deal about it. . . . He was a wonderful Bible student and knew many stories from the Bible." A friend wrote of him: "I have always thought of Jim as a combination of wisdom, wit and the joy of living and a deep religious understanding of humanity." Polly Plesset speaks of the "genuine religious faith" of both James and Ruth Waring. Although Ruth and he belonged to the Church of the Ascension (Episcopal) at East Sixth Avenue at Gilpin Street, he was not a regular churchgoer. Always mindful of his need to replenish his energy level, he used Sundays as a day of rest.

Like his students, Waring's patients remember his sense of humor. Long before Norman Cousins, former editor of the *Saturday Review,* healed himself of a painful illness by watching funny movies (as related in *Anatomy of an Illness*), James Waring used humor as therapy. His lightheartedness was a balm for his patients. Lucile Harrington closed her letter with a postscript: "I don't wish you to think our friendship was all serious. We were attending a TB meeting in Rocky Mountain National Park. Dr. Waring called my husband and asked him if he was wearing a black tie; he had just seen a man pass by wearing a tuxedo. Mark answered that the man was a waiter."

He liked to quote Satchel Paige, the baseball player—"If your stomach disputes you, lie down and pacify it with cool thoughts," or "Don't look back. Something might be gaining on you." He told stories and jokes, was whimsical, and could be a tease. And that is what stayed in patients' memories about him, along with his competence and compassion—his ability to make them laugh.

Lucile Harrington, in recounting her remarkable story, concluded: "Dr. Waring's picture hangs in our study, and I look at it every day. He, with the love and encouragement of my husband [who is no longer living], is the reason I am alive and well at 84."

And what about Waring as a patient himself? "Nurses loved him," recalls Dr. J. Cuthbert Owens, who performed minor surgery on Waring. "He praised and complimented nurses." "'Bring Dr. Waring back as much as you can,'" he recalls their saying. Furthermore, says Owens, he never had a "brushfire" following him, as often happened with other doctors, which he attributes to his "rapport, good judgment and insight in dealing with others."

Waring showed an interest in Nu Sigma Nu, a medical fraternity, lending money to start the local chapter. (Later the members gave a prize in his name, making him one of three doctors so honored.) "The Patient and the Physician" (1950) is a revision of the Nu Sigma Nu address Waring delivered at the University of Colorado School of Medicine on May 17, 1949. Some advice he gave the future physicians:

> In the presence of the patient no remark should ever be made that might conceivably add to his anxiety and apprehension. Never forget that he is watching you like a hawk for the slightest sign of hope or hopelessness. . . . Restrain all expression of pleasure over some sign or symptom. . . . Elation over some interesting pathologic sign cries to high heaven that you have lost sight of suffering humanity. Pure compassion is ingrained and cannot be taught, but outward expressions may mean nothing more than thoughtlessness.

Dr. Thomas Petty, a chest physician, educator, and one-time director of the Webb-Waring Lung Institute, putting it simply, says that Waring's greatest interest was the patient with diseases of the chest, not "chest problems." "Dr. Waring's fundamental interest was in patients and their welfare."

11 New Assault on an Old Disease

IN JUNE 1946 Waring went to Saranac Lake, prudently taking long underwear; he remembered how cold and rainy it could be, and it was. He had dinner with Francis Trudeau, son of Dr. E. L. Trudeau, and visited the sanatorium. He wrote to Ruth on Hotel Saranac stationery, which had underneath the hotel name, "Modern—fire proof—European Plan" and below, in equally bold letters, "Tuberculosis Patients Not Received." A statue of Trudeau had been placed at the sanatorium in 1918. The sculptor was Gutzon Borglum of Mount Rushmore fame. Engraved at the base of the monument were the words of the adage held in such high regard by Trudeau, and by James Waring as well: "To cure sometimes . . . to relieve often . . . to comfort always."

Then Waring went to Buffalo for a medical meeting devoted to the new drug streptomycin, which appeared to be effective in controlling tuberculosis. "It is thrilling to see and to hear what it does in animals," he wrote Ruth, "so far [it is] toxic in some human cases. Need to find out what these effects are." It was his nature to be cautious, despite being as impressed by the drugs as others were.[35]

Streptomycin was discovered in 1944 by Selman Waksman, a Russian émigré working at Rutgers University. A soil microbiologist and marine bacteriologist, he isolated more than eight substances he termed "antibiotics." D. H. Corwin Hinshaw, M.D., of the Mayo Clinic conducted a trial of streptomycin against tuberculosis and had encouraging results. With the advent of chemotherapy for tuberculosis, a new era was being ushered in, one which few could have foreseen at that early date.

From the late 1940s onward James Waring was in the forefront in the trials of chemotherapy for tuberculosis, using streptomycin, para-aminosalicylic acid (PAS), and later isoniazid in carefully controlled studies. Responding to a call from the surgeon general of the United States, Waring collaborated with Lt. Col. William H. Roper in a follow-up study of thousands of military patients who had been discovered to have minimal pulmonary tuberculosis or pleural effusions. Financing for the study came from the U.S. Office of Scientific Research and Development. The papers coauthored by Drs. Roper and Waring on tuberculous pleurisy are still considered landmark papers on this subject.

Among the centers where the change in therapy was taking place was Fitzsimons Army Hospital, which became a major tuberculosis and chest disease facility. Located in Aurora, a suburb east of Denver, the hospital was built in 1917 as a tuberculosis sanatorium. In November 1945 approval was given for an arrangement with Fitzsimons whereby members of the Colorado General Hospital staff might act as civilian consultants, enabling the army hospital to be approved for residency training.

The study of minimal tuberculosis had actually begun as early as 1944, with Waring as responsible investigator; Col. George F. Aycock and Col. Esmond Long (longtime director of the Henry Phipps Institute in Pennsylvania and James Waring's friend) as consultants; and Lt. Col. Roper as director of the section. For at least five years, 141 young males in military service were observed. "Primary Serafibrinous Pleural Effusion," published in 1952, stated that in young adults, "acute serofibrinous pleurisy with effusion of the type here discussed is practically always tuberculous in origin."

Of the patients processed in 1947, the first year that streptomycin was widely used, 1,932 were treated on the Tuberculosis Service, 403 of whom took part in chemotherapy research. From 1947 to 1956, the first ten years of such studies, 14,380 patients were processed in the Tuberculosis Service, and most received chemotherapy. Maj. Gen. C. W. Tempel, M.C., retired (formerly chief, Department of Medicine, and commanding general of Fitzsimons Army Hospital), and Col. J. A. Wier, M.C. (later commanding general of Fitzsimons), in 1964 wrote of this postwar period: "Dr. Waring's help with this unusual case load was immeasurable. He pioneered the use of tuberculosis chemotherapy, and ultimately chemotherapy alone in order to cure disease. . . . His lectures at the hospital were always concise and informative." Students, they wrote, were charmed by his warm, intimate manner.

Dr. Roger Mitchell, who would become director of the Colorado Foundation for Research in Tuberculosis, met Waring at Fitzsimons during the war. "He was the consultant to the Tuberculosis Service at Fitzsimons, at which time there were 6,000 patients there, and I was just one of those 6,000," Mitchell said at the Waring symposium in 1963. "I remember that he had the time to come and see me and talk to me, which very much impressed me." It was a propitious first meeting, for a little over a decade after their meeting the by then well-qualified Mitchell would turn out to be just the man needed in Denver.

When new methods for treating chest diseases were being tested, Waring was one of the national leaders supporting them. He kept abreast of the various surgical procedures and was an advocate of resectional surgery, where indicated, with the new chemotherapy.

"Until 1945," according to Mitchell, "the chief specific treatment was collapse therapy, in which an infected lung was collapsed and put at rest by artificial pneumothorax, effected by introducing air between the lung and chest wall; or by thoracoplasty, in which a permanent collapse was induced by surgical shortening of the ribs; or phreniclasis, or the crushing [temporary paralysis] of the phrenic nerve." These measures were designed to make the lung occupy less space temporarily or permanently, and thus close cavities, reduce multiplication of the tubercle bacillus, and enable healing to occur. Dr. Michael Lubchenco remembered that Waring "disliked thoracoplasties, which he considered a deforming procedure."[36] He also opposed the removal of residual scars after adequate chemotherapy. Writing in 1960 to Dr. H. McLeod Riggins, he reminded him that he had voiced caution about "pimplectomy," the removal of residual lesions after a short period of treatment of active pulmonary tuberculosis. "I am sure you and I have seen many of these cases get well without surgery and remain well thereafter," Waring wrote. "Furthermore, if in days gone by these residual lesions in many, many instances remained healed, it would be logical to expect that after proper chemotherapy the chances of relapse would be still less." According to Dr. Burns Amberson, Waring's scorn for the procedure led in some degree to its being discontinued.

In 1954 Waring told the Minnesota Tuberculosis and Health Association: "Lung surgery expanded, especially lung resection, after it became clear that chemotherapy prevented postsurgical tuberculous complications. . . . In due course, it became evident that the preoperative chemotherapy was so effective that surgery was seldom necessary."

James Waring changed his views on bed rest. Quoting John Hunter (1728–1793), a Scottish surgeon—"Don't ask me what I said yesterday! Ask me what I think today!"—he wrote in 1954 about the trend toward chemotherapy and less rigid bed rest. "For some patients, bed rest destroys morale, instigates rebellion, defeats purpose. Leads to uncontrolled boredom, restlessness." Another area in which Waring changed his mind concerned side effects of antibiotics. He wrote in 1948, when streptomycin had not long been in use: "Experts agree that deafness is not a serious or frequent toxic effect," then changed his opinion about the drug because of vestibular damage, which causes loss of balance; this turned out to be a serious side effect and was one of several reasons research continued. Another disadvantage of streptomycin was that the tubercle bacilli tended to become resistant to it. In 1946 PAS was developed, and in 1949 it was used in combination with streptomycin. Isoniazid, which had been synthesized many years before, in 1952 was discovered to be effective against tuberculosis. Isoniazid used with streptomycin or PAS proved to be the best combination. Finding the most effective dosages and sequences was the long-awaited breakthrough.

Dr. W. H. Helm, who met Waring when he was a visiting professor at Brompton Hospital in London in 1954, in a letter to the author provides a glimpse of Waring's showmanship:

> He enjoyed telling a true story about a Veterans hospital treating tuberculosis with streptomycin, which in those days had to be combined with the nauseating but important para-aminosalicylic acid to prevent bacterial resistance: suddenly bright coloured streaks appeared staining the whitewashed outside walls of the hospital—each streak just below the window above a bed and due to a chemical reaction between the drug and the whitewash as the soldiers dispatched the horrible liquid to the world outside as soon as the nurse's back was turned. During a lecture at the Brompton Hospital Dr. Waring took great delight, and to the amusement of the large audience, in demonstrating this reaction with materials provided for him by the resident medical officer.

A tradition began in 1952 when Waring asked his former student, John Durrance, to organize an internal medicine postgraduate review conference. It was held three days before Labor Day at Estes Park, Colorado, in the mountains northwest of Denver, a convenient site for a congenial gathering of physicians to discuss chest cases. First known as the Estes Park Chest Conference, and then from 1958 as the James J. Waring Chest Conference, it was sponsored by the Colorado section of the American Trudeau Society and was organized along the lines of a "consecutive-case presentation conference."[37]

These conferences and similar ones organized across the nation were the first Physician Standard Review Organizations (PSROs) in the United States. Comparisons were made of various forms of therapy for tuberculosis, including bed rest, diet, climate, collapse therapy, surgery, and chemotherapy. The forum was, as one doctor has described it, "an honest baring of soul, in order to more carefully audit what we are doing in the practice of medicine. It is of immense disciplinary and teaching value." The conference was given a special flavor by the "El Toro" session. Durrance had begun these sessions at the Denver Veterans Administration Hospital, where he was chief of the Chest Service. These Friday afternoon teaching conferences attracted unusual cases from the city. "It was a game," says Durrance. "Give a person only an X ray with just the date, name, sometimes birth date, left/right sides. 'What do you see? Want the history?' A lot of private physicians came to the VA. Lots of fun, sometimes cruel." As described by Dr. Melvin Johnson, a regular participant for many years, "Half the time it was something wild: Jack Durrance—in fact, everyone—loved to trick people."[38]

Waring brought distinguished doctors to the chest conference, such as his old friend, Dr. J. Burns Amberson of Columbia University. One year, two physicians came from abroad whom James Waring had met in 1954 when in England—Sir Kenneth Robson and A. F. Foster-Carter, both pulmonary consultants of Brompton Hospital, London. As Johnson tells it, he and Durrance picked up the British doctors at the airport.

"Jack always had a big car and was a fast driver. He got them on the Virginia Canyon Shelf Road [to Central City]," noted for being only one lane, very steep, with a steep dropoff. "Foster-Carter sniffed snuff, presumably to calm his nerves. He'd never seen a mountain over 600 feet high before."

Attendance at individual sessions averaged from thirty-five to forty persons. Old programs in Dr. Robert K. Brown's collection provide an excellent overview of the subjects considered. Doctors from several facilities that served Indians in the region attended through the years. The conference addressed such issues as patients leaving the hospital prematurely against medical advice, interrupting treatment, and not restarting treatment until in a moribund condition. Although tuberculosis was the main disease considered, many other chest diseases were discussed, including silicosis.

Brown states: "There was fascinating material from the Rosebud Sioux Reservation and from New Mexico. After the second year of the conference we always had one segment on TB in Native Americans. People would come from as far as Alaska who had treated Eskimos and Indians from the north with TB."

Beginning in 1961 a similar gathering called the Midwinter Chest Conference was held in March in Aspen, Colorado. (Yet a third conference, the Aspen Emphysema Conference, also known as the Thomas L. Petty Aspen Lung Conference, met each June.) The Midwinter Chest Conference, which had become known as the John R. Durrance Conference, merged in 1989 with the Estes Park chest conference, and the combined meeting, held in Aspen in March, is now called the James J. Waring–John R. Durrance Chest Conference.

FOLLOWING the death of Gerald Webb in 1948, Waring, an associate research director for a quarter century with the Colorado Foundation for Research in Tuberculosis, was elected president and research director. He was still professor of medicine when he accepted the positions.[39] He further followed in Webb's footsteps in April of that year when he was elected an associate editor of the *Annals of Internal Medicine,* the official journal of the American College of Physicians. He also served as examiner for the American Board of Internal Medicine's subspecialty of pulmonary diseases. To Ruth he stated: "The Board of Internal Medicine I will have to work with but it will come easier for a number of reasons." He continued to serve as a consultant to Fitzsimons Army Hospital and to the Veterans Administration.

James Waring was particularly moved when in March 1949 he received the Alfred Stengel Award of the American College of Physicians "in recognition of his many years of loyal and devoted service to the College, his outstanding influence on medical education and his contributions to the practice of Internal Medicine and Clinical Research." He had long recognized the importance of membership in medical societies that brought doctors together and provided a forum for academic presentations. A tribute to Waring after his death, published in the *Bulletin of the School of Medicine* of the University of Colorado, cited another advantage: "The happy cosmopolitan atmosphere of our Medical Center is due, to a great degree, to the efforts of Waring to bring to the School distinguished visitors from all parts of the world. This was no mean accomplishment in the pre-jet era when Denver was somewhat remote. He could do this because of his personal acquaintance with the greatest medical talent of his time."

The collegial atmosphere kept the doctors at the medical school abreast of changes in the field. The trend at the medical school was toward subspecialties. In the 1950–1951 catalogue, the following divisions of the Department of Medicine are listed: internal medicine, neurology, dermatology and syphilology, industrial medicine, and general practice. New research efforts were launched in the area of cardiac disease. Dr. S. Gilbert Blount came from Johns Hopkins to head a cardiac catheterization laboratory. At the same time, Dr. Henry Swan in the Department of Surgery, with help from Dr. Robert Virtue, anesthesiologist, was developing a new technology for operating on the heart by using hypothermia, or cooling of the body. With the development of open heart surgery, Drs. Swan, Blount, and Virtue brought national and international attention to the medical school.

In 1951 Darley brought in as chairman Dr. Gordon Meiklejohn, a virologist from the University of California School of Medicine. The following year, Waring retired from teaching in the Department of Medicine in the summer of 1952. He would be sixty-nine that year, and retirement age had been fixed in 1936 at sixty-eight. Waring would relinquish part of his teaching duties but would continue to attend patients of Colorado General Hospital and fulfill his duties connected with the Colorado Foundation for Research in Tuberculosis.

James Waring was now professor emeritus. With the changes occurring in his professional life, it was a time for taking stock of the years. Family stories were often in his thoughts. A few years earlier he had shared some family history in "The Family Circle" (1949), delivered before the American College of Physicians. He told about an ancestor, Dr. Francis K. Huger, who in the early nineteenth century was "adventurously involved in an abortive effort to rescue General Lafayette from prison in Austria" prior to the French Revolution. He introduced Theodosia—daughter of Aaron Burr, vice president of the United States—who married Joseph Alston (later governor of South Carolina) and may have died at the hands of pirates. Waring traced his ancestry to the Alstons; Thomas Pinckney Alston, his great-grandfather, was a half-brother of the governor. The episode had caught his—and his listeners'—imagination, providing a departure from the usual medical meeting fare.

Another paper, "The Physical Examination: Helps and Hindrances" (1948), became a classic for its good sense and humor. Waring's colorful language made an impression upon a generation of medical students—he spoke of examining "the lady over forty summers . . . below abdomen to umbilicus: trespass at your peril!" Allen True illustrated the paper with whimsical drawings. What better testimonial to the power of a paper than this recollection offered by Dr. Herbert Rothenberg, a Denver internist:

> I took my Internal Medicine Boards, which still had the orals, at San Francisco General Hospital in 1958. There was an elderly patient in a large ward. I took a history—he had a chest problem—

> and I did a physical exam: nonspecific abnormalities. I had no clear-cut idea of what was wrong with him. I looked at him more closely; the room was relatively dark. . . . I remembered that not long before I'd read an article by Dr. Waring on how to conduct a physical exam. A major point was [the necessity of] adequate light.
>
> There was a long window shade, floor to ceiling, pulled down. I pulled the shade and the roller came down and hit the patient in the head! It split his scalp! I called for the nurse, who brought a suture tray and I sewed up the laceration. . . . .Then, done, I took a look in the good light. I saw his face and shoulders were cyanotic; this told me that he had superior vena cava obstruction. It made the difference between my passing and failing.

In 1953 Waring was given the Trudeau Medal by the National Tuberculosis Association (NTA). The medal was first awarded in 1926. Dr. Burns Amberson, in charge of the chest service at Bellevue Hospital in New York City from 1938 to 1955, gave the main address. He, too, had contracted tuberculosis, and he became one of Waring's closest professional colleagues. Although a little older than Amberson, Waring said he would like to be known as "one of Amberson's boys." Dr. Julius Wilson of the University of Pennsylvania wrote that in the field of tuberculosis Drs. Amberson and Waring "were giants indeed but never rivals, although their lives were parallel because all were engaged in the same organized fight against tuberculosis."

Two warnings were sounded at the meeting. Held in Los Angeles—with the largest attendance ever—the gathering attracted more than 2,000 physicians, nurses, and other public health workers who wanted to learn about the new drug therapies. One warning was that Americans could not hope to feel safe from tuberculosis because the disease was rampant in many of the less-developed countries of the world and increasing travel and contacts with the rest of the world could affect them. The other was that treating ambulatory patients with the new drugs might result in "vast reservoirs of drug-resistant organisms in partially 'cured' individuals."

Waring was pleased to see his friend Mark Harrington made president of the association, only the third layman to hold the position. At the Waring symposium, Harrington noted that in 1943 Waring had persuaded him to head the Denver Tuberculosis Society, although he had done no work in public health before. Harrington stated:

> Some years after that, the Society decided that we needed a good

> health department in this city which did not have one at all in those days. . . . We finally were able to persuade the mayor to consider the possibility of having a complete survey made of the health conditions of the city. . . .
>
> I went away for a time to acquire a group of investigators who would be competent to make this study. While I was away, the powers that be called Dr. Waring downtown and told him that if he would withdraw his support from me, they would be willing to see to it that a new health officer was appointed who was a doctor (the previous one was not). Dr. Waring, however, refused to let me down. . . . Never, in all of our long association, did he ever ask me once to do something that I thought wasn't the right thing to do.

Harrington was referring to the part he had played in Denver's postwar health planning. In 1944 Governor John Vivian appointed Dr. Florence Sabin chairman of the subcommittee on public health. She was seventy-three and had retired from the Rockefeller Institute for Medical Research in New York City, where she had studied blood cells and vessels, lymphatics, and bone marrow. Tuberculosis was another interest, and for two decades she worked with the NTA Research Committee, integrating the tuberculosis studies of private and government-supported institutions. With a grant from the Commonwealth Fund, Dr. Carl Buck of the American Public Health Association made a careful study of the vital statistics of the State Health Division and then made recommendations for correcting inadequacies. A subcommittee was formed to study the report and to draw up bills to be presented to the legislature. The result: eight measures, known as the Sabin Health Bills.

The subcommittee's next task was to tell the people of the state about Buck's report, which meant traveling all across the state. Sabin visited all sixty-three counties, even paying all her own expenses. The medical society gave up its tax-exempt status so that it might lobby to support the health measures.

Waring supported their efforts, particularly their fight against tuberculosis and undulant fever (Bang's disease), a disease of cows spread from dairy herds. Although the measure regulating dairy standards passed, the measure to provide a sanatorium for tuberculosis patients—which Waring long had advocated—was defeated. Instead, a new tuberculosis ward at Colorado General Hospital was authorized. Overall, six of the eight measures passed, which was considered a resounding success for the health of Colorado. The so-called cow health bill (referring to Bang's disease) was defeated but passed in 1948.

James Quigg Newton, Jr., who was elected mayor of Denver in 1947, made public health a special interest. Quigg Newton won the largest vote of any mayor in the history of the city up to that time. In what was a departure from Waring's usual distance from politics, he took a personal interest in the candidate, whose wife Virginia was the daughter of his old friends, the Morrison Shafroths. In 1954, when Newton ran for the U.S. Senate, Waring sent money to his campaign, writing: "He has brought about a transformation in our public health situation which many do not know about or appreciate." Ultimately defeated in the Democratic primary race, Newton served as mayor until 1955 and in 1956 became president of the University of Colorado.

In 1953, Sabin died. Waring had admired her courage, determination, and effectiveness in working for the betterment of health in Colorado. At services at St. John's Episcopal Cathedral on October 5, 1953, he was an honorary pallbearer. The nation had lost a distinguished scientist; he had lost an ally, a fellow bibliophile, a patient, and a friend. When Waring was given the Florence Sabin Award in 1955 he was greatly honored that an award in the name of this gifted physician, who had accomplished so much in public health and medical research, should come to him. Mark Harrington was asked to present the award, and among his words were these: "Whether it was popular or unpopular, professionally expedient or inexpedient, likely to succeed or fail, make friends or provoke enmities, he [Waring] has always been willing to stand up and be counted for what he thought was right."

Two years earlier, the Colorado Conference on Tuberculosis Workers had created a James J. Waring Award, given annually to the person who contributed most to tuberculosis control in Colorado. Ironically, that person may still have been Waring. He continued to speak out on anti-TB measures all over the country. He recommended frequent X-rays from early childhood on and annual x-rays for every man over forty and every woman over forty-five. In March 1955 he cited these TB figures: one million cases in the United States; 250,000 known active; 200,000 undetected, 86,000 new cases in 1954; 12,500 deaths in 1954.

Waring still believed that sanatorium treatment supplemented by chemotherapy was best for the tuberculous patient. In his 1954 address to the Minnesota Tuberculosis and Health Association, he said: "Sanatorium treatment for tuberculosis patients has by no means been replaced by modern chemotherapy. . . . It is the best place for the patient to stay while he gets well, and it provides isolation that prevents the patient from spreading his disease to others. . . . I am fearful that the quick improvement of so many patients under chemotherapy may delude both patient and doctor into thinking the disease is cured when it is only asleep, and carriers of communicable disease may be returning to their homes with disastrous consequences to both relatives and friends."

The pendulum was swinging away from sanatoria, however. Most tuberculous patients could be maintained by chemotherapy on an outpatient basis, leading to the closing of sanatoria. For example, Swedish National Sanatorium in Englewood, a Denver suburb, became Swedish Hospital in 1956. Name changes proliferated in the 1950s. Reflecting the new era, the subspecialty of tuberculosis changed its name to "pulmonary disease."

Although preventive inoculation against tuberculosis, in which live but weakened tubercle bacilli are used as a vaccine, had been introduced in 1921 in France by Albert Calmette and Camille Guerin (Bacillus Calmette-Guerin, BCG), it would be two more decades before the vaccinations gained appreciable acceptance in the United States. A significant disadvantage of the BCG inoculation was that the recipient always tested positive thereafter. The procedure did not gain extensive acceptance in this country until after 1940. Waring advocated use of BCG vaccine in the late 1940s and 1950s. It was effective, he believed, if a live, well-proven vaccine was used.

Children were of particular concern to him. J. Arthur Myers, M.D., in an article in *Journal-Lancet* (1964), wrote of Waring's interest in long-term studies conducted on children and his participation "in a study which consisted of a complete examination of infants. These examinations were repeated periodically as far into adulthood as possible. He wanted to observe how initial invasion with tubercle bacilli behaved when acquired at different ages in the lives of children and young adults."

Long a champion of the tuberculin test, Waring believed that the proof of infection it furnished, if administered early enough, played a vital role in combatting the disease before it had progressed dangerously. In "The Current Treatment of Pulmonary Tuberculosis" (1954) he wrote of the two important functions of the tuberculin test: first, telling if tuberculous infection had taken place or not; and second, telling "when that infection took place and even where that infection occurred."

In 1955 Waring joined the Committee on Tuberculosis of the American School Health Association and became enthusiastic about the certification of schools program. Using as his forum the association's meeting in Milwaukee on May 21, 1955, he spoke on "Achilles Heel of Tuberculosis Control": "The weak spot of our enemy, tuberculous diseases, is its curability in its early stages. Its strong point is its capacity for multiplication by virtue of its contagiousness. Ignorance and delay in diagnosis inevitably results in one person with open tuberculosis infecting one or more persons and so on ad infinitum." He called the tuberculin test "the most important diagnostic tool available for any infectious disease." What could be simpler? "When the test is positive, the person harbors a tuberculosis focus somewhere in the body." His charge to the association: "Find the early case, cure it with chemotherapy, prevent it from becoming a spreader of disease." The Achilles heel was on the foot of the doctor who did not perform the tuberculin test: "It is as simple as guinea pigs and dandelions! This multiplication has got to stop!"

Part Six | *Final Years*

12 *The Family Grows*

IN THE SPRING of 1945, following Anne's graduation from Wellesley, she and Ruth took courses at the University of Pennsylvania. "We lived in an awful apartment," Ruth says of this period. "Drunks across from us, noise, windows breaking, cockroaches." But there may have been value in the experience. When visiting them in Philadelphia in May 1946, James wrote Ruth: "The girls are learning certain things there which are mainly self-reliance and social adjustment. . . . You and I can only suggest gently—not dominate—and pray over them."

The sisters soon moved back to Denver. After an interval of studying painting and design—interests she has followed with a passion through the years—Anne began working at Graland Country Day School. There she was asked to be the school's first librarian. She later taught reading, history, arithmetic, and science. In the summer she continued her volunteer work as a nurse's aide in various clinics at the medical school.

Ruth, meanwhile, took a job in the Division of Industrial Hygiene at the School of Medicine. Jane McGilvray, a co-worker, says Ruth was a "true researcher," but Ruth did not like laboratory work. Her interest turned to occupational therapy, and she went to Mills College in Oakland, California, as a graduate student. While visiting her Uncle Will Porter at his winter residence in Riverside, she met Robert Halpenny, who followed her when she went to a rehabilitation center in Santa Monica. After a three-week whirlwind courtship, they became engaged. On January 11, 1950, Ruth married Robert in St. Martin's Chapel of St. John's Episcopal Cathedral in Denver, with a reception at 910 Gaylord Street. The bride was happy that it was a small wedding but says it was more formal than she would have preferred: "Robert wore spats!"

They settled in Riverside. The family rejoiced in December with the arrival of their first grandchild, Ethel Waring Halpenny. A grandson, James Robert, followed in 1952. Grandfather Waring's joie de vivre was irrepressible: In 1952 he wrote to his wife, who was visiting the Halpennys: "Just about ready to jump on my horse and gallop (or is it Gallup) (what is your opinion)—well, as I was saying—canter off in all directions, me 'orse being Yellow Taxicab Tabor 5151 or something like that. Will view house (now but a hole in the ground) before I go."[40]

This happy family news helped offset other, less fortunate events. In 1948 Antonio had suffered a heart attack, and his health steadily deteriorated. In the summer of 1951 he spent five weeks in a hospital in Boston, where he was diagnosed and operated on for gallstones. On August 19 he wrote, "I have been well and cordially treated, no small part of which I owe to my brother—somebody asked me if I was the famous Dr. Waring. I said, 'No, just his brother and proud of it!'"

It was one of the saddest days of James Waring's life when his brother died in January 1952. They had been extraordinarily close and owed much of their happiness and success to the support each had given the other in childhood and throughout their lives. Antonio had carried out to the letter his mother's admonition, written when he learned he had made Phi Beta Kappa at Yale: "I want you to cultivate a steady cheerfulness, a persistent healthy outlook, a large sanity of view and a warm-hearted thankfulness." Antonio Waring was revered in Savannah, not only for his medical care and for the time he devoted to the health center clinic but also for his interest in civic improvement. As chairman of the Park and Tree Commission, he had worked to preserve historic landmarks, especially the handsome squares. He thought the city should expand rather than sacrifice the unique city plan and recreation areas.

When James Waring received a letter in 1953 saying that the alumni association of Lawrenceville, his prep school, wanted to note his being awarded the Trudeau Medal in *The Laurentian,* he wrote: "It is of much more interest that my brother, Antonio J. Waring, of the class of '99, was head boy of his class. I lost this brother two years ago and do not recall that I saw any notice in *The Laurentian.*" He sent the association clippings telling of Antonio's many accomplishments.

Waring was extremely proud of Antonio's sons, Antonio Jr. (Tono Jr.) and William (Will), who both had done well in medical school. To his brother he had written in 1942, "I am very happy to know that young Tono graduated second in his class. He is a fine boy." Antonio Jr. later took time from his practice in Savannah to follow a longtime interest in archaeology. William Waring became a member of the faculty in the Department of Pediatrics (and later, head of the department) at Tulane Medical School in New Orleans. His wife, Nell-Pape Williams, is also a physician.

Antonio Sr.'s daughter Anne and her husband, Mills Lane Jr., a banker, went deep-sea fishing with the Warings in the 1950s. Maintaining close ties with family was important to Waring. Always interested in young people, he helped them when he could. Dr. John Lunt, his old friend Lawrence Lunt's son, says Waring helped him to get into medical school. "He gave me some of his archaic medical tools and his black bag. . . . He was one of the world's special people and I loved him."

Lawrence Lunt wrote to say that he was "deeply touched and moved by your giving [John] your medical bag." During the war Lawrence Lunt had flown coastal duty with the Civil Air Patrol. At war's end he and his wife moved back to Colorado to search for a suitable ranch. During that year they lived at The Farm and saw a lot of the Warings. The Lunts settled on the Double-Four Ranch in Wheatland, Wyoming, and Waring visited them there fairly often, enjoying fishing and the comfort of time spent with old friends. Sometimes Anne and her mother went also, along with Porch, Anne's Springer spaniel. Following one of their visits Lunt wrote: "Every time I go up to the mail a few minutes late, the mail-carrier has come and gone. Often when I go a little earlier, he is late. So it was this morning; he has broken a fan belt and was an hour behind his usual schedule. Were it not for the milk I wouldn't have waited, but come back to see you and Anne off. But milk, you know, is the River of Life on a milk-dry ranch, so I could not leave it up in the hot mail box to sour on us. Milk, like myself, sours too easily!"

As more friends bought land there, The Farm became a compound. Dr. Mason Morfit, a surgeon who arrived in Denver in 1948, tells about his own acquisition: "I was looking for a place to build a house in the country. Waring had sixty acres, the Waring Farm. I bumped into him in Florida, fishing. I asked him if he ever planned to sell and he said, 'This morning at breakfast, Ruth and I decided to unload our unworldly possessions. Drop your hat where you want it.'"

The Farm continued to bring much pleasure. It was lent on occasion to organizations such as the Faculty Wives Club of the medical school, and the Warings entertained faculty, old friends, and visitors there. A continuing tradition was the Fourth of July party. One of Ruth's social clubs, the Wednesday Music Party, met at The Farm in the spring for "The Road Show." Held in the playbarn, it provided an opportunity for the participants to don costumes and perform funny songs and dramas, sometimes involving husbands. Ruth delighted in joining in, easily encouraged to perform on the nose flute or sing in the chorus. She insisted the group be called "the party" and not "the club." She and longtime members "Dickie" (Mrs. Cyrus) Boutwell and Margaret (Mrs. Roblin) Davis never missed a meeting of the Wednesday Music Party. "Ruth lived by the rules. 'That's not the way the bylaws were written,' Ruth was likely to say at meetings," a friend says. "She couldn't relax the rules; she lived her life that way." The group had been formed in 1906, and Ruth had belonged to it since its beginning.

Jeanne Erskine, musician and fellow "party" member, tells of returning folding chairs to storage space under the stairway after the Wednesday Music Party's Christmas program:

> After parties I remember helping to put these back in a particular order. Christmas carol books had a special shelf. Ruth was a superb party giver and organizer who loved to join with friends in farce and fun, skits and stunts. . . . Behind the scenes things were always planned so that everything fell into place; guests felt welcome, well-fed, and comfortable.
>
> I remember Christmas times especially. The Denver families and their children who had grown up together had a Christmas Eve party at the Warings'. . . . We [she was then Mrs. Basil Reeve], along with the Mitchells, the Filleys and other new medical school associates were invited. Dr. Waring was a merry host, always a story teller. . . . 'This man was riding along, d'you see . . .' I can hear him now—a charmer."

In August 1953 the Warings moved to their newly built house on Hawthorne Place. Considerably smaller than 910 Gaylord, it still was spacious enough to accommodate such gatherings as the Wednesday Music Party's annual Christmas party and the Warings' Christmas Eve party, which continued to be held each year with the old circle of friends.

Two weeks before Christmas in 1954 the Halpennys had another child, William Stuart, and Christmas Eve provided a second cause for celebration: Anne's engagement to Edward D. White, Jr. White recalls: "Anne in those days tended to wear squaw dresses from Santa Fe and wear moccasins or go barefooted around the house and at parties [with her contemporaries]. Jim called the guests together—Shafroths, Tolls, Emerys, Blickensderfers, Swans and other old Denver friends, plus medical people—and said: 'I've always believed that someday the right man would catch up with Anne and put shoes on her. And now that has happened.'" White was then introduced and the engagement announced. Anne and Edward had planned to marry in June 1955 after he graduated from the School of Architecture at Columbia University, but the wedding was postponed because of the illness of his father. Waring explained the situation to a friend:

> Unfortunately, he died following a serious operation in late July. This cast a little gloom over the prospects of a wedding in Denver. Since Mrs. Waring and I had planned for a vacation in Jackson Hole, Wyoming, and since Ruth and her husband and their three children had planned to meet us in Jackson, we shifted all the plans to Wyoming and Anne and Ed White were married in a lovely little church in Moose, Wyoming [on the Snake River, just outside of Jackson Hole]. Had a little wedding reception at the ranch where we were staying and the owners of the ranch very kindly turned the place over to us for a family wedding dinner. One of our good friends had to stand guard at the gate to the church in order to keep two bus loads of tourists from intruding during the ceremony.

Anne and her father had always been especially close. After his death a friend wrote, "I can remember casual moments in the last years since [we] came to Denver when something you said or did made it crystal clear to me how much and in what a special way you loved him." Others have commented as well on the very special bond between father and daughter.

Waring was at ease with young people in general, and many felt close to him. On countless occasions he wrote letters on behalf of young people to help advance their education or their careers. Dr. Kenneth Robson, an English acquaintance, told Paul Anderson of Waring's trans-Atlantic telephone call to enlist Robson's aid in enrolling a friend's son in a school in London. Ranald MacDonald, Anne's contemporary, shared a vignette showing Waring's natural rapport with the younger generation: "How delightful of him, for example, when one day Pam and I were invited to lunch and I was about to disembowel a squab on the plate before me, to hold up a restraining hand and say, 'Hold on, Ranny. I am in a pious mood today. I feel like saying grace.' And so he did. The squab was delicious."

"OH, TO BE IN ENGLAND . . ." How often must James Waring have thought this, with his interest in English history in general and English medical history in particular. Invited to be a visiting lecturer in chest diseases and to give a paper at a medical symposium at Oxford, he accepted—once he had convinced Ruth that they both should go. To Sue Waring, his brother's widow, he wrote, "'The Little Woman' has, somewhat reluctantly I fear, finally capitulated and says that she will go with me."

In March of 1954 he wrote his cousin J. Frederick Waring, who had written a family history, asking him to send information about the activities of their grandfather, James J. Waring, and great-grandfather, Dr. William R. Waring, during their respective visits to Britain after medical school. Frederick had taught at British schools in the 1920s before returning to teach in this country. With his usual thorough ways Waring boned up on British history and kept a journal. He read his account into a dictaphone for transcription by his secretary. The result is a typewritten, seventy-four-page, single-spaced account of the people he met, the cases presented to him, the sights he saw, and the traditions he observed.

Writing to his English cousin, Hilda Coleman: "I have received an invitation from the Brompton Hospital to visit London to take part in the teaching program for the months of June and July. . . . I have also been invited to give a paper at the annual meeting of the British Tuberculosis Association at Oxford in July."

They sailed from New York on the *Nieuw Amsterdam,* May 21, 1954. His English colleagues arranged things so that he had time for sightseeing as well as medical visits, and Ruth had invited a Denver friend, Mrs. Robert (Mary) Barkalow, to come along so that they could sightsee when Waring was occupied with medical affairs. His first visit to Brompton Hospital, the world's first general chest hospital and a leader in modern pulmonology, came on June 1.[41] "Act natural but not too natural" was the warning he had received from his friend, J. Burns Amberson of Bellevue Hospital in New York, about visiting Brompton. "Never have I received better advice!" he wrote a friend soon after his first visit. "Even at this moment I am struggling more or less unsuccessfully to heed it."

Happily, Dr. W. H. Helm, a registrar, or chief resident physician, was assigned to be his "personal assistant" while Waring was in London. In the journal he is described as being "a very fine, attractive, most helpful young man." When shown the doctor's lounge at the hospital, Waring was delighted to see pictures of famous physicians associated in the past with the hospital, but his joy was short-lived. In his diary he told of "a doctor entering the lounge (with whom I am to make rounds next week). . . . Dr. Helm remarked to him that I seemed to have a remarkable knowledge of the famous men whose pictures were hanging on the wall," to which the second doctor remarked that "'they had made very little or very poor contributions to medical knowledge.' This remark . . . I thought was highly scandalous. I all but told him so."

Waring noted that many of the hospital's doctors were the sort of people he liked: well-educated, very curious, and lively clinicians. He thought Brompton Hospital very clean, tidy, well ventilated, and attended by fine nurses, doctors, and residents. "I was very favorably impressed," he wrote.

Waring kept copious notes on all the patients he saw, visiting men's, women's, and children's wards. He wrote of the case of an epileptic girl who had a cavity, negative sputum, and no tuberculin test; he thought the cavity might be due to her having aspirated vomitus into the lung during a seizure. He added in a margin note: "She had a negative TT [tuberculin test] later! I was right."

He gave his first lecture of the trip on June 2 on "Current Chemotherapy of Pulmonary Tuberculosis" to one hundred doctors. The next day he was taken to Arlesey Sanatorium, forty miles out of London, where he saw x-rays of Norwegian refugees, "curious shadows extending out from the roots of the lungs on both sides." These men had rowed across the North Sea and developed amazingly powerful pectoral and back muscles, which cast shadows, making x-rays hard to interpret.

After both Warings visited Frimley Sanatorium in Surrey, they visited Windsor, observing the boys at Eton in their morning coats, white ties, and striped trousers. They were especially impressed by the evening service at St. George's Chapel at Windsor Castle, more properly called the Chapel of the Knights of the Garter.

Waring lectured on pleural effusion on June 9. He commented in his journal that "British doctors are so convinced that practically everybody shows a positive tuberculin test that they don't use it very often. . . . I pointed out that the tuberculin test under these circumstances was of the greatest possible value in differential diagnosis whereas in our country where there are so few persons with a positive tuberculin test that a positive tuberculin test there was correspondingly of considerable value." A letter to the author from Professor Scadding:

> At [the time of his visit] the academic activities which the Hospital had undertaken in a rather informal way for many years were being given a more formal setting by the establishment of the Institute of Diseases of the Chest as part of the British Postgraduate Medical Federation, a school of the University of London; and we invited Dr. Waring, as a much respected physician in our specialty, to visit the hospital and its developing, postgraduate institute. . . . I remember him as a scholarly, dignified, outstandingly courteous figure.

> At the end of his visit, he gave me a copy of his edition of MacMichael's "Gold-Headed Cane," which I am pleased to have still in my library.

On June 9 Waring spent the afternoon "with Mr. [Russell] Brock, the famous British surgeon[42] who is today more of a surgeon in cardiology than he is a pulmonary surgeon. . . . Showed me a number of interesting cases. . . . I liked very much Mr. Brock's attitude towards [a patient]. . . . the fact that he examined each patient himself using the stethoscope freely. He laid great stress upon the importance of wheeze and I showed him Gerald Webb's maneuver of listening with the stethoscope at the [patient's] mouth in order to hear a noise."

And what better city for a bibliophile than London? He took Ruth to Marks' Book Store, 84 Charing Cross Road, and bought a present for their friend, Jack Durrance, an iris expert: *The Genus Iris.* Throughout the diary, Waring made constant notes of "books that I should get."

Dr. Kenneth Robson, who acted as a host while Waring was in London, took him to two clubs, one being the Athenaeum, founded in about 1830 and known as "The Club of the Literati." Portraits of Charles Darwin and Thomas Huxley graced the lobby. Robson, in a letter to Paul Anderson, stated that Waring's tenure as visiting professor at the Brompton Hospital made a great impression on the staff and students there. He recalled that while discussing a patient with disseminated tuberculosis who had been presented on ward rounds, "Dr. Waring made the impressive aphorism: 'In disseminated tuberculosis, the victory is gained or lost in the lungs.' Dr. Waring's rounds, and his aphorism, were long remembered in that hospital."

During the postwar period, the Warings sent care packages to his cousins, Hilda Coleman and Elise Molyneux, and had the opportunity to meet Coleman on June 13. She lived at Carlyle Mansions on Cheyne Walk, between Cheyne Row and Lawrence Street—which is where Henry James passed the last four years of his life, Waring noted in his journal.

A black-tie dinner at the Royal College of Physicians on June 17 gave Waring an opportunity to witness a ceremony that the historian in him relished. He described having his name announced by the toastmaster as he arrived, then meeting the aptly named president of the college, Sir Russell Brain, a distinguished neurologist. First came a toast to the queen, and then the introduction: "'Me Lords and Ladies, Fellows of the Royal College of Physicians, Ladies and Gentlemen: The Queen.'" Waring's account continued:

> While we were sitting in a rather small room where the lecture was to be given, only about 100 or 150 people to be accommodated, the audience suddenly became quiet and everybody rose to their feet and the procession of the president and his four assistants and the speaker all filed in, preceded by a footman in livery carrying a huge mace. The huge mace was then put with a smaller scepter, which the president of the College carried, on a large red cushion beneath the desk where the speaker was to give his lecture. The president of the College then stood up and addressed the audience with the simple statement that Dr. Livingston would now give the Mitchell lecture. Dr. Livingston then, robed in a beautiful red robe, went up onto the platform and gave his lecture. When he completed the lecture, the footman took the huge mace off the red cushion, handed the scepter to the president and with the mace leading the procession, followed by the president and his four assistants and the speaker, Dr. Livingston, they all filed out through a door. . . . After they had left, the audience then dispersed.

The following evening he went again to the college as a guest of Robson for the medical committee's dinner for the Hospitals for Diseases of the Chest. Dr. Maurice Davidson, who knew of his interest, brought Waring a book—much to his delight—containing an essay by Sir John Forbes called "Happiness and Its Relation to Work and Knowledge," dated 1850. His diary entry: "The menu included four different wines and brandy and Scotch whiskey. After dinner Dr. Kenneth Robson brought me home"—and then, in red ink, "(Sober! I swear!)."

He was taken to visit St. Bartholomew's Hospital, founded in 1123 in a section of an Augustinian priory. His notes burst with enthusiasm, noting paintings on the walls, minute details. He told of William Harvey, discoverer of the circulation of the blood, appointed physician to the hospital in 1609. The earliest record of a medical school being there dates from the year 1662. The names of some doctors are cited, and in the margin of his diary he wrote, "Caneholders." Much of "St. Bart's," as it is commonly called, was destroyed in World War II, "but they had moved to Cambridge during the war." Missing among all the details in his journal about St. Bart's was any reference to his grandfather, James J. Waring, who had served there as assistant resident physician just over one hundred years before.

And so it went in London: visiting hospitals, lecturing, making rounds, and attending social events with doctors, interspersed with vigorous sightseeing and note-taking on historical subjects that caught his fancy. An entry on the origins of the fortune that launched the Tate Gallery: "Henry Tate, founder, was grocer's boy, entered sugar business and invented 'Tate's sugar cubes.' No one had thought of this before."

An emotional and intellectual high point of the visit to Britain came for Waring when, at the Royal College of Physicians, he held the original Gold-Headed Cane: "The president of the College, Sir Russell Brain, was good enough to take out of its precious case the Gold-Headed Cane and sent word to me among the group that he wanted me to see it as I had expressed interest and I again had the privilege of holding it in my hand and inspecting it. The head is of gold with the coat-of-arms of wearers arranged around the head. The shaft is probably malacca." He also noted that the cane's age was "approximately 134 years."

On June 22 at Brompton Hospital he gave his fourth lecture, this time on "The Surgical Treatment of Pulmonary Tuberculosis," and on the last day in June delivered his fifth lecture at St. Thomas's before the entire Brompton staff. The next day, at the London Chest Hospital, discussion concerned a doctor who dealt with patients with asbestosis, twenty of whom had developed cancer of the lung. An alarm was just beginning to be rung about this disease, but it would take many years before the dangers were fully recognized.

Dr. W. H. Helm, who did such a good job of shepherding Waring to chest hospitals in London and its environs, described his recollections thirty-five years after Waring's visit:

> This is just how I remember Dr. Waring—a slight, elegant, scholarly, courteous, very gentle man. He was an excellent listener who would let me run on and then chip in with an observation which would enhance the subject and inform the talk, in a most unobtrusive way. He had wide interests but especially in medicine and medical history and a very nice sense of fun and humor. . . .
>
> I remember only one rather discordant episode which occurred when I arranged for him to meet a senior physician who was quite a pioneer in certain aspects of chest medicine, and who was a good friend of mine, but who, quite unknown to me, harboured some sort of resentment against visiting American physicians, who he seemed to think were coming over here to tell him how to do his job. This attitude and his naturally fiery temperament led to a most uncomfortable quarter of an hour during which the gentle philosopher James J. Waring remained charming and under complete control of

his emotions, only releasing them in a whispered hiss as he parted from the belligerent physician, "That man's a bully."

A surgeon took him to the Wye River to fish. He recounted in his journal: "It is a perfectly lovely spot. . . . We walked down the hill about 100 feet to the road, crossed the road and then down about 50 feet to where the river flows. At this point the river was fast and the water heavy and the fishing obviously dangerous. Within an hour I had hooked a large salmon but found it very difficult to move up and down on account of the rapids and the rough shore and the slippery rocks. After about twenty minutes my salmon got away. This was the only fish I hooked that afternoon." The next day they fished "very arduously but we failed to catch anything or ever to hook a fish." But he had a wonderful time.

Waring wrote of "a very satisfactory visit at the Chelsea Physic Garden with the curator, a Mr. Mackenzie," on July 24. Mackenzie showed him around the grounds, took him to the laboratory "where research is being carried on on plants and showed me the books and the old library. . . . Here was the first, or one of the first, seed exchange systems among the botanic gardens of the world."[43]

Now it was time to travel. The Warings hired a car and drove first to Oxford, departing on July 4. The annual general meetings of the British Tuberculosis Association took place July 7–10. Lectures were held at the School of Geography of Oxford University. When Waring gave his talk on "The Pathogenesis and Prognosis of Tuberculous Pleural Effusion" on July 9, leading British pulmonary physicians were present, as well as guests from other countries. Sir Clement Price-Thomas, "the very dynamic Welsh surgeon whom I had met in London," amused him by saying that "the thoracic surgeons were really nothing more or less than demolition squads." Waring told his journal that it seemed a very appropriate term, "since the surgeon was called in to clean up a serious mess after a lung was pretty well shot to pieces."

Next they journeyed to Wales and as far north as the Lake Country of England. Waring not only saw the sights and made notes about the towns they stayed in but also visited hospitals and met doctors. In Wales they visited Wrexham, the town in which Elihu Yale, the founder of Yale University, was buried. Yale was born in Boston in 1649, returned to his father's homeland to spend the final decades of his life and died in 1721, Waring wrote in his journal. He agreed with the comment in an article on a descendant of Yale that "The history of Ial (the old

Welsh word for Yale, coming from the basic meaning of 'useful in the spiritual, intellectual and material senses') is not confined to a man, a family, a university, a town or a province, but in reality is the history of a nation, the cymry, the brotherhood of Britain and America."

A plaque in Lincoln Cathedral had this inscription: "These western transcepts and the Central Tower were restored 1924–30 by Albert Farwell Bemis in loving memory of his mother, Alice Cogswell Bemis, born at Ipswich, Massachusetts, January 5, 1845, died at Colorado Springs, Colorado, October 18, 1917." In his journal he wrote, "This Mrs. Bemis, a friend of my mother and Bemis Hall at Colorado College."

After their tour of England, the Warings returned on the Olympia in early August. For Waring it had been one of those wonderful interludes when life had a connectedness, with special meaning on professional, intellectual, and emotional levels.

13 | *A New Role*

WHEN Waring stepped in and took over the leadership of the Colorado Foundation for Research in Tuberculosis, the program needed revitalization. The death of Gerald Bertram Webb in 1948 came two years after another severe loss: the death of Dr. Charles Boissevain, the foundation's first research director. A chemist and bacteriologist, Boissevain had been a major investigator for over twenty years. After he returned from duty with the Army Medical Core, he had concentrated all his efforts into finding a mold that would inhibit growth of the tubercle bacillus. In the process he discovered two molds of the genus ***Fusarium*** that had this property. Dr. Florian Cajori, professor of biochemistry at the University of Colorado School of Medicine in Denver, began further study on the antibiotic substances produced by the molds. Dr. Mary Alice Hamilton kept the laboratory in Colorado Springs going during the war and at the time of Webb's death was serving as associate director. Little was being done now, however, in the laboratories.

Waring recognized the importance of locating the foundation on the Denver campus of the University of Colorado School of Medicine, which offered the advantage of proximity to experts in the fields of physiology, biochemistry, and pathology. The trustees shared this view and urged him to negotiate with Dean Darley and other university officials regarding the transfer of the foundation's laboratory work to the Denver campus. Waring was authorized to develop plans for such a transfer, and in 1949, with the support of university president Robert Stearns, an affiliation agreement was voted by the regents of the university. The National Tuberculosis Association awarded a grant to further the foundation's work.

The medical school had a space problem, so it was necessary to build a separate building for the foundation's laboratories. The trustees of the foundation were responsible for providing the architectural plans for the new building, subject to the approval of the university, and for raising funds for its construction. Terms called for the university to own the building and rent it to the foundation in exchange for services for fifty years (until the year 2002), with the option to renew for another fifty years. Land at the southwest corner of the medical school adjacent to the Florence R. Sabin Research Building was set aside for the new building.

Members of the foundation research staff were given faculty appointments in appropriate basic or clinical medical school departments, but the new facility had its own board of trustees and endowment funds. The university alliance provided a distinct advantage in fundraising: Philanthropic foundations promised to contribute $75,000 if private donors would provide the remainder of the estimated $150,000 cost of the building. Waring took personal responsibility for raising the necessary sum; he and Ruth made a substantial contribution as an initial gift to the project.

The cornerstone was laid on April 22, 1953, by Joel A. H. Webb, a son of Gerald Webb. Among the contributors were the El Pomar and Bemis-Taylor foundations in Colorado Springs; the Barth, Boettcher, Bonfils, Lawrence Phipps, Van Hummell–Howard, and Johnson foundations in Denver; Vincent Youmans's Tuberculosis Memorial Fund, New York; Glockner-Penrose and St. Francis Hospitals, Colorado Springs; the Estate of Charles J. Denison; various tuberculosis associations through the sale of Christmas seals; and many individuals.

The venture took courage on the part of Waring, who wrote a friend, "I signed a contract for this building, and personally committed myself when we were still shy $5,000 to meet the initial cost of construction and an additional $20,000, at least, for moving into the building and for additional equipment and furniture."

Contributions were generous, and the target figure was reached. Within a year of ground-breaking, the two-story, 5,000-square-foot building was completed. It would support additional stories, to be added later as needed and when the money could be raised. The foundation would not take in patients; it was to be devoted to research.

Dr. René Dubos, microbiologist and pathologist at the Rockefeller Institute in New York City, was the principal speaker at the building's dedication, March 12, 1954. He spoke on the chemotherapy breakthrough. With words from Descartes' *Discours,* "Fac et Spera"—Work and Hope—as its motto, the same words Webb had chosen thirty years before, the foundation had constructed the building without cost to the university. Waring said the foundation's $250,000 endowment fund remained untouched and would be used to finance research in the new building's laboratories.

The foundation's work expanded rapidly, and Waring soon felt it was time for him to relinquish his position as research director of the facility to a younger man, someone who also would teach in the medical school. It so happened that he knew just the man for the job—the director of the Trudeau Sanitarium, which had recently closed. A graduate of Harvard Medical School and Waring's one-time patient, Dr. Roger Mitchell was a leading authority on tuberculosis and other pulmonary diseases. He had experience in university teaching and had had a private practice.

In 1955 Mitchell became director of the foundation and also had charge of the tuberculosis wards at Colorado General and Denver General. He brought with him from Trudeau his friend and colleague Dr. Giles Filley, a clinical physiologist. J. Carroll Bell, M.D., and Howard D. Olson, Ph.D., also were on the staff.

In his first report as director, Mitchell told of waning interest in tuberculosis research as a result of the improved treatment in this country, although the disease remained a scourge in many countries. He suggested that the word "tuberculosis" be removed from the foundation's title in order to increase attractiveness to good researchers. He would, in fact, push for a name change for the next five years.

Waring, as president of the board, wrote in his report for 1955–1956, "Although our dominating interest is research in tuberculosis, certain other important disabling disorders of the lung are under study." Then he launched into a subject about which he had strong conviction: "An unfortunate, even dangerous, impression seems to prevail here and there that tuberculosis is licked! This is far from the truth. Since 1947 the death rate for tuberculosis has fallen dramatically, but the number of those sick with tuberculosis has not decreased in proportion. . . . New drugs and brilliant surgery are saving lives but they also are prolonging the lives of many patients who do not make perfect cures but continue as more or less chronic invalids, often as an infectious menace to their contacts." In 1957–1958 he reiterated this theme: "Despite 'miracle' drugs and dramatic surgery, tuberculosis is far from being a conquered disease. Tuberculosis accounts for more deaths than all the rest of the infectious and parasitic diseases combined."

Olson resigned in 1956, but two new recruits strengthened the foundation: Alfred J. Crowle, Ph.D., microbiologist and immunologist, and M. Laurance Morse, Ph.D., geneticist, joined the staff. "This laboratory is bursting at the seams," Waring wrote to Dr. Esmond Long in April 1958. "The boys are pressing me to add two more floors to the building. I am out 'beating the bushes.' Hope that I can 'flush' a little money from here and there."

It was a period of phenomenal growth for health research, both in public and private support. The Health Resources Facilities Act of 1956 established a program of assistance to provide essential improvements or additions to existing and needed facilities, as well as matching grants for construction of research facilities nationwide. The foundation received a grant-in-aid from the U.S. Public Health Service in 1958 to help put on another floor to the laboratory. Grants also were coming from the National Science Foundation and the National Institutes of Health. The third floor was completed in 1960. Meanwhile, in 1959 Oscar K. Reiss, Ph.D., joined the laboratory staff as head of the foundation's Division of Biochemistry. As part of its research, the division would investigate the normal and abnormal chemical reactions that occur in lung tissue. Drs. Reiss and Waring became good friends. Two years later the trustees again were under pressure to add two more floors despite the addition of the new floor.

In 1959 Crowle, appointed assistant professor of microbiology in the medical school and head of the foundation's Division of Immunology, began work on developing an antituberculosis vaccine. The closest thing to an effective vaccine was the useful but flawed Bacillus Calmette-Guerin (BCG). Although funds for research in general were increasing rapidly, funding for tuberculosis research in particular was dwindling. "Chemotherapy was in full swing," Crowle observes, but "TB became resistant to drugs." He would continue his work on experimental vaccines.

Mitchell continued pushing to rename the foundation to reflect the change in emphasis to a broader spectrum of diseases, but Waring wanted to keep the emphasis where it always had been—on tuberculosis. Following a continuing dialogue between Drs. Waring and Mitchell, in 1959 the foundation was renamed the Webb Institute for Medical Research, with the subtitle, "Dedicated to the Study of the Diseases of the Lung." With the aid of Filley, the research concentration shifted from tuberculosis to chronic obstructive pulmonary disease (COPD). Filley was also especially interested in the function of breathing.

In his president's report Waring clarified the name change: "Name change does not mean a change of purpose. This laboratory was set up for the study of tuberculosis primarily but not exclusively. . . . [It is] desirable that we should enlarge our interest in certain other very important diseases of the lungs, notably emphysema and chronic bronchitis."

In 1959 Ruth Waring gave money to the foundation to set up the James J. Waring Chair of Biology: M. Laurance Morse, Ph.D., became the first occupant of the position. Morse recalls that in about 1961

Waring became "aware of the fact that molecular biology was coming into medicine and would add a great deal to medical research and treatment of patients. Waring clearly recognized [the importance] of basic considerations."

UP UNTIL HIS DEATH, Waring was spending half a day at the institute, pushing himself and inspiring others, propelled by the importance of the center's work. Florence Sabin believed it was a disadvantage to set a retirement age. "People age at different times and I'm sure idleness doesn't contribute much to happiness," she is quoted as saying. "We've got to remain active and interested in ideas. That's the way to keep young." James Waring kept young in mind and spirit through involvement: teaching, supporting the Webb Institute, seeing patients, writing and helping others with their writing, exchanging ideas, and, perhaps most of all, continuing to learn. "Have met new men and learned some new things," he wrote Ruth from a medical meeting. A colleague observes, "The characteristic that made him Jim Waring was his enthusiasm, as he continued always to be a student in search of additional knowledge and truth."

A vignette from his paper "The Gentle Doctor" (1955), illustrates the contagiousness of his love of learning:

> Late one afternoon in the Denison Library, I was looking up something; the student assistant brought me a journal. He quickly discovered what I was interested in and I found myself shortly well-nigh surrounded with other references for which I had not asked. More than that, I presently found him on the other side of the table, reading and doubtless digesting and retaining better than I, everything he had fetched from the stacks. Somewhat overwhelmed, I said, "It's getting late! Don't bother any more." To which he replied, "But, Dr. Waring, I want to learn what you are learning." I caught him by the ears and kissed him on both cheeks! The librarian finally had to throw us both out!

Dr. George Bower, a former resident, says of Waring, "It never ceased to amaze me how he kept abreast of things in so many fields, far removed from his primary interests in medicine." Laurance Morse tells of how Waring asked him to find books to read about new developments in science. Waring wrote to a friend in 1959 that he and Ruth were taking lectures on chemistry and physics. These were on television, in the early morning and evening. "I have been delighted with what I have heard. I have learned quite a little bit. The lectures are rapidly reaching far beyond me I fear . . . we have listened to some 40 of these lectures."

He did not dwell on the aging process. Although he spoke of his life expectancy, he rarely mentioned his own specific infirmities, and when he did so, it was usually in a joking manner. Yet he continued to show concern for the maladies of others. When he learned that Harriot Hunter Jardine's brother, George, an artist in Los Angeles, would have to have his arm amputated because he had developed a sarcoma of the right shoulder, Waring wanted to help however he could. She was, she recalls, "at wit's end" after talking to several doctors about her brother's situation. "Let me work on it," Waring told her, and through his network of friends and colleagues, he contacted someone at the Veterans Administration in Los Angeles who had developed a shoulder girdle prosthesis. The prosthesis enabled her brother to go back to work teaching art and made his final months productive and brought him satisfaction. James Waring had never met George Hunter, but he cared and he acted.

"In [Dr. Waring's] declining years, I admired his tenacity and continuing professional involvement in every possible way," wrote Dr. J. Philip Clarke in an appreciation in *History of the Department of Medicine.* "He, of course, was involved in the new Webb Institute. But he was always available to provide consultative advice, still anxious to present scientific papers even when he had to labor to climb the steps to the podium due to his own progressive pulmonary insufficiency."

Waring's interest in semantics persisted. He had acquired a reputation as one concerned with the correct usage of words and was generous with his time, helping others who asked him to look over a paper, a chapter, or give other advice. Sometimes it was just a question of a single word: President George Norlin of the University of Colorado once wrote a long letter to him about the use of the word "syndrome," saying that he would prefer "syndromy."

Dr. Alfred Crowle, professor of microbiology of the Webb-Waring Lung Institute, recalls:

> I remember that when I gave him a draft of my book, *Immunodiffusion* [published in 1961], for comment and criticism, he was especially concerned about phrases and words. For instance, we had a several-minute discussion about "miniaturize," which I used in my book. He argued very persuasively that I should use "miniatured." His stance was of a classicist and scholar; mine was that language

> is a dynamic vehicle—he probably would have replaced "dynamic vehicle" with "evolving tool." I am sure that many of today's "-ized" words would grate on his linguistic sensibilities. But he would also accept—and from time to time use—them with a gracious bow to "progress." He was a stickler for proper English usage.

"Acquire the habit of looking things up, promptly! Don't delay! Let the cakes burn! . . . Look that word up now!" he urged in "The Gentle Doctor," his speech at the first annual banquet of the Alpha Omega Alpha chapter at George Washington University, 1955.[44] He sprinkled puns generously throughout his papers and his talks, spicing up scientific papers with Waringesque phrasing: "All the catgut in Christendom or kittendom" or, in another, "bug and buggage." He would spare no effort in pursuing a good pun. In 1956 he entered into correspondence seeking information about Nathaniel Bowditch, who traveled in a one-horse chaise from Salem throughout New England, with great improvement of his tuberculosis. The correspondence resulted in the inclusion in his Amberson lecture, "The Chest Service at Bellevue Hospital: A Better Mousetrap" (1956), of a memorable line referring to Bowditch's trip as the first authenticated history of "chaising the cure."[45]

A colleague spoke of his "shock-producing words," a reference to his unorthodox language in medical papers and talks. On May 26, 1956, Waring delivered the first Amberson lecture at the annual meeting of the National Tuberculosis Association and its medical section, the American Trudeau Society. Admitting that giving his talk "without emotion I find difficult because my heart is over there with him"—Amberson was abroad and unable to be present—Waring continued:

> To avoid outward display of emotion one may say or do strange things. I have in mind the story of the bereaved widow of a miner killed in an accident. A committee of miners went to call on her. When she appeared in the door of her little cabin with face contorted with grief, they offered her a bunch of flowers and lamely tried to say a few comforting words. After swallowing her Adam's apple a few times, she burst out with, "Go to Hell! Me heart is broke."

On many occasions, Waring said that the University of Colorado was his school, so he was especially moved when the honorary degree of Doctor of Science, honoris causa, was conferred upon him by the university in 1956. Another honor came his way the following year, when a tablet was erected at Denver General Hospital to commemorate the achievements of Drs. Charles Elder, G. W. Holden, and James Waring in the field of public health. Johns Hopkins bestowed upon him the Fifty Year Alumnus Medal in 1958, although he had not actually graduated from that institution. Waring subsequently wrote a letter to the president of Johns Hopkins University, Milton S. Eisenhower, in which he said that he felt troubled about accepting the medal because he was not a graduate of the university. He offered to return the medal. The president graciously declined the offer, writing that if Waring was willing to acknowledge his relationship to Johns Hopkins University, he would honor the University by keeping the award.

In 1961 Waring was named one of two American fellows of the British Thoracic Society, known today as the British Thoracic Association. The Royal Society of Health and the British Tuberculosis Association also conferred honorable membership upon him. To a student he said: "I always think that a pat on the back during a lifetime is worth much more than a large bouquet of flowers on your grave. Somebody has said that under these circumstances you can't smell the flowers."

Few pats on the back could have touched James Waring more than having a student society named in his honor whose purpose was "to stimulate broad interest in the art, history and philosophy of medicine . . . in an atmosphere of informality and conviviality." The establishment of the Waring Society at the University of Colorado School of Medicine was a tribute of which he was especially proud.

The origins of the Waring Society can be traced to a meeting between Ben Eiseman, who was then associate professor of surgery and chairman of surgery at the Veterans Administration Hospital in Denver (affiliated with the medical school), and Roger Wotkyns, a third-year medical student. The two were talking one day in 1954 about academic performance in college. Wotkyns, a member of Alpha Omega Alpha (AOA), thought selection to the honorary medical society was arbitrary: real scholars, he said, would not necessarily be those chosen for AOA. The academic selection process, he believed, involved more, and he was particularly concerned about including those who had clinical research as their goals. Eiseman told him about Harvard Medical School's Boylston Society, in which membership was based not on academic achievement alone but also on personality. The society had been in existence since 1811, and its bylaws—with which, as a former member, he was familiar—provided a model for the type of society that both men envisioned.

They talked with Waring about their idea of a society similar to the

Boylston, to be named the Waring Society. The professor emeritus got up and left the room, and when he reappeared, apologized for his abrupt departure.

"Please forgive me," Waring said, "I needed some time to compose myself." "He was tickled," Wotkyns recalls.

At the time of their visit, Waring was ill and they tried to cut the meeting short, but he was enjoying the conversation. Finally, Ruth Waring—who had learned to assume the position of "watchdog" where her husband's frail health was concerned—had to step in to contain her husband's enthusiasm and graciously saw to it that the visitors left.

The other organizer was another student, Jim Weaver. Membership was to be limited to fifteen juniors and fifteen seniors "who demonstrate unusual interest in the aims of the Society." Each spring, five members of the sophomore class were elected by the membership; others were chosen the next fall.

"James Waring epitomized intellectual stimulation, joie de vivre. He liked young people," Eiseman says. When he wrote to Waring, sending him a certificate of the Waring Society, the professor emeritus responded, "Boy, am I really set up!! I really am very proud. . . . I really think it should have been called the Ben Eiseman Society." A constitution was drafted and approved in February 1955, and the society was named for Waring on March 3, 1955. It was officially recognized by the medical school in June 1955. At each meeting a paper was read by a senior member on any subject of his or her choosing, approximately forty-five minutes in length, followed by discussion. Cash awards were given for the two best papers each year; these were submitted to the *Rocky Mountain Medical Journal,* and some were published.

Eiseman states: "Their papers were written entirely without reference to any course requirement and largely without direct faculty direction. They thus reflect a commentary of what the brightest and best of the medical students were thinking about their chosen profession of medicine during their student years. It is no wonder that members of this society went on to make contributions in medicine in the years following graduation—just as did the alumni of the Boylston Society at Harvard."

The high point of each year was a meeting at the Warings' home. "Always there was Dr. Waring's inimitable wit," says Eiseman, "and his delightful recollections of his early mentor, Dr. Osler, of early days in Colorado, of trout fishing, and of the growth of the University of Colorado School of Medicine. He held the meeting in his house every year until the last year of his life, even though he had to rest in bed for a day or two before and after the meeting. Mrs. Waring knew how much this meant to him and allowed Dr. Waring the indulgence. To the very end Dr. Waring sparkled with wit, erudition and stimulation at this cherished annual event for the society."

In the Waring Room in Denison Memorial Library of the University of Colorado School of Medicine are several bound volumes of papers presented before the Waring Society. An early paper, "Man's Changing Patterns of Thought as Reflected in His Attitudes toward Disease" by Fred J. Julian, advised that "The study of the ancient evidences of disease is known as paleopathology. . . . It is interesting to note that the skeleton of this man, Pithecanthropus erectus, shows what is the earliest record we have of disease in man—a marked exostosis of the left femur. Altogether, there is a remarkable record of bony disease in fossil man, including rickets and Pott's Disease [tuberculosis of the spine]."

In view of his visit to Britain in 1954, Waring would have been especially interested in a paper by Alice R. Bishop, "The Great Men of Guy's—Their Work and Their Hospital." Prompted by a visit she had made to Guy's Hospital in London in 1955, she wrote: "As I stood in the courtyard of this hospital and in the very rooms where so many famous men had stood and worked since its beginning, history began to live for me and all the people of whom I had heard and read and whose names I had used so unthinkingly became real and I was a part of it all."

Her respect, in refreshing contrast to the blasé young doctor he had encountered at Brompton Hospital, would have delighted Waring. She spoke of Sir Russell Brock, "who lectured to us last year and will probably be best remembered for his quotation, 'The heart is a pump and not a music box.'" Most likely Waring had issued the invitation to Sir Russell to visit the medical school when they had met the year before.

A prize paper, presented in 1957 by William E. Jobe and David K. Hills, "The History of Medical Education in Colorado," would have been of special interest to Waring, as would the "Best Paper" the following year by Watson Bowes, "The Knight of Norwich," about the life of Sir Thomas Browne. Bowes told that Osler "often admitted that Browne was his life long mentor. . . . In 1868 at age seventeen William Osler purchased his second book, the 1862 edition of *Religio medici* and when in 1919 Osler's body lay in the chapel of Christ Church College, Oxford, this same copy was placed upon the casket." James Waring would have been touched to see that a student shared his reverence for both men.

Some of the members came to feel close to Waring. He shared with them his Christmas 1907 letter from Trudeau and told them of his own self-pity and of the frustrations of that bleak period in his life. Dr. Thomas Petty, a Waring Society member who graduated in 1958, recalls, "He was very friendly and warm, rarely threatening. A spellbinder. He made everything interesting."

A tribute to Waring appeared in the *Rocky Mountain Medical Journal* of May/June 1979 by Petty, in which he told that during his tenure as president of the Waring Society he asked if he might bring "a certain fermented malt beverage." Waring sternly warned him that such libation was not allowed in the Waring home and no such frivolity would mark any meeting of that society which bore his name. Later, when the members arrived, "there was spread before them a magnificent spread, fantastic snacks, and the beverage of choice." After the paper was presented, they retired to his library for reminiscences and relaxation, and it was then, Petty recounts, that he recognized by the subtle twinkle in Waring's eye that he had been "playing me like a fish that was about to be released."

PETTY'S METAPHOR was an apt one, for fishing was Waring's favorite means of relaxation. "The angler practices his art in an ideal setting of pure air, lovely scenery and silence. At best only nature's voice speaks in his ear," he wrote. But fishing was much more than a sport for him; it was a bridge to others, just as it was a chance to commune with nature and a game requiring skill and the use of one's wits. He was able to fish, despite his physical limitations, because he would nap or rest alternately with his morning and afternoon sessions.

Every summer he put aside time to spend fishing with family members and friends in streams and lakes of the West and, occasionally, the Gulf of Mexico off the Florida coast. Antonio came every summer from Savannah to spend time with James, and the brothers fished at various mountain resorts, such as the A Bar A Ranch near Encampment, Wyoming. He was devoted to fly fishing and liked to send flies and leaders to various fishing cronies. Waring went salmon fishing in Canada, bonefishing off the Florida Keys, pursued high adventure on the North Fork of the Snake River near Jackson Hole, Wyoming, and pursued steelhead trout on the Rogue River in Oregon. He also fished with friends in the Wigwam Club near Deckers, Colorado, and in the "Fishing Friends," organized by Robert Sayre, a mining engineer. Then, to his great joy, his wife took up fishing in the 1950s and became an enthusiast, too.

"The mere catching of fish is a sterile affair," Waring said in his presidential address to the Clinical and Climatological Association at

Skytop, Pennsylvania, in October 1941. "But the fisherman who sallies forth in the true spirit of Izaak Walton, with ear attentive to the voice of nature and eye observant of her wonders, will return from his expedition with a renewal of that strength which is a magic compound of body and spirit."

Waring pasted to his copy of *Daily Strength for Daily Needs,* which he kept by his bedside and referred to frequently, a verse by William Neder:

> God grant that I may live to fish until my dying day.
> And when it comes to my last cast I then most humbly pray
> When in the Lord's safe landing net I'm peacefully asleep
> That in His mercy I be judged good enough to keep.

Waring's other great hobby, book collecting, continued to bring him joy. "Fortunate is that man in whom love of good books is ingrained. . . . Great persons of yesteryear will gather at his elbow," he wrote in "The Gentle Doctor." "Love of good books is contagious. . . . Prescription: an inquiring mind, an eager concern to get knowledge, a quality indispensable in a doctor, anyhow."

Because James Waring enjoyed books so much, he wanted to share them. His enthusiasm for books went far beyond the bounds of medical history, for he enjoyed a wide range, including poetry, early western history, science fiction, and the classics. The staff at Pooh Corner Bookstore in Denver knew his reading preferences and brought him new volumes on favored subjects. He sent a book about William ("Buffalo Bill") Cody to Dr. René Dubos of the Rockefeller Institute for Medical Research. Dubos, born in France, was enthralled, and his reply to Waring tells of "the influence of tales of 'The Wild West' on the concept of America in my generation of Europeans. . . . In reality the important aspect of the book is to make clear that for the world at large Buffalo Bill soon became the symbol of an immensely exciting moment in human history."

But when it came to lending books, Waring liked to be sure he would get them back. Dr. Roger Mitchell says he was the fortunate recipient of several texts from Waring, but admits, "I was guilty of keeping books too long two or three times."

By 1950 Waring had begun to accelerate his donations to medical libraries. Yale University received several books.[46] The Beinecke Rare Book and Manuscript Library of Yale also received contributions from Waring. According to the librarian of the Beinecke Library, these books number eighteen, most of which concern Galileo. When he was a student at Yale, Edward D. White III, a grandson of Waring, saw these impressive handwritten manuscripts and was told that it was "the largest Galileo collection in one place."

As James Waring had been led to collecting by others, he encouraged those around him to start their own libraries. He helped Dr. George Bower start collecting when he gave him an old dictionary. "I have been a dictionary 'nut' ever since," he confesses, "as well as a book collector. Waring supplied me with names and addresses of antiquarian medical booksellers and I was able to quickly get into the hobby of collecting." In 1961 Waring sent him a warning: "I hope your wife realizes that you are becoming a bibliophile. I hope your enthusiasm does not result in the children going barefoot. The risks are great."

Waring took an interest in establishing and personally designing a medical history reading room in the Denison Memorial Library at the medical school and donated funds for its completion. The original Waring Room, which no longer exists today,[47] is said to have been beautifully appointed with wood-paneled walls and furniture picked for comfort as well as utility. He began giving books to Denison Memorial Library prior to his death, hoping to encourage interest in the history of medicine; the trend in medical school curriculum was to do away with courses in that subject.

In 1954 Malcolm Wyer, librarian emeritus of the Denver Public Library, assessed a Waring collection presented to the library. "The most distinctive feature of the collection is the group of books by and about Laënnec," he said. "Such a collection could be gathered only by persistent searching of book catalogues and book stores extending over many years and could only be duplicated today with great difficulty and at heavy cost."

When Gerald Webb died in 1948, his family gave his library to the medical school. His collection, which included some rare volumes on chest disease—with some valuable Laënnec editions, including a reprint of Vesalius' *Fabrica* from the original wood plates—was placed in what was at that time the faculty reading room of the Denison Memorial Library. The combined Webb and Waring collections are considered one of the world's most comprehensive sets of rare volumes on chest disease, with Laënnec, so revered by both men, their focal point.

Following Waring's death, Malcolm Wyer gave Ruth Waring an appraisal of her husband's library:

> It is unusual for one man to show a keen interest in books on so many different subjects as are found in this library. . . . The medical

> collection contains approximately 800 volumes and a considerable number of pamphlets, reprints, etc. There are over twenty-five editions of *The Compleat Angler* by Izaak Walton and about 400 volumes in the Limited Editions Club, non-medical classics such as Shakespeare, Tolstoy and Dickens.

Ruth Waring donated 935 of these books to the Denison Memorial Library in 1964. She also donated his large collection of reprints from medical journals, the oldest dated 1866.[48]

In addition to his collection of books, Waring had a large collection of reprints from medical journals, many in French or German. Included were more than 300 from *Annals of Medical History,* followed in number by the *Bulletin of History of Medicine.* Favored subjects were Galen, Jenner, Harvey, Hippocrates, Hunter and, of course, Laënnec. The oldest reprint, dated 1866, was on "Ventilation." Most in the collection, however, were post-1930. He also had a fine collection of medical cartoons and prints.

Waring's great love for knowledge—be it in the form of books, clinical research, or student papers—never faltered. He maintained it even in the final chapters of his life.

14 | *Undaunted*

AT A MEDICAL MEETING in St. Louis in 1957, when Waring was seventy-four, he became ill with pneumonia and had to be rushed to the hospital. As he described it months later, he was "put in oxygen, filled up with hip shots that raise h-e-l-l with my colon, and managed to survive both the pneumonia and the antibiotics but have had a difficult time getting my strength."

After returning to Denver, he was troubled by shortness of breath. He wrote another friend that the illness had "left me with a laboring pump" and a "leaky arteriosclerotic valve," and that his activities were very restricted. "It has left me more or less a lame duck. I can waddle, but only very slowly." He was bothered by Cheyne-Stokes respiration, and his doctor told him that he had symptoms related to altitude but that if he were careful and took medication and oxygen daily and did breathing exercises, he could continue to live in Denver. He wrote to the doctor who'd taken care of him in St. Louis that he was better, but still short of breath. "I still keep a tank of oxygen beside my bed, however, and if I am restless and troubled by periodic breathing, I resort to it and find it very helpful."

Those who knew James Waring better noted a change, however. Polly Riedeburg Plesset says he "became concerned about his own mortality. As he became older, he was more apt to be ill. I think it frightened him. He had so much more knowledge [of the disease process]; he'd had so much illness." But this was a private side that he showed to few. Dr. William Millett, son of the Warings' neighbors and friends, the Daniel Milletts, also noticed the change in Waring, commenting on his concern to his wife Alice.

But Waring refused to let illness take over his life—he had too much to finish, too much to live for. On September 28, 1957, Anne presented her parents with their fourth grandchild, Edward D. White III, who became known first as Teddy and later as Ted. Anne says photographs of her father holding the baby show his love and joy but also his frailty and weariness. Despite his failing health, Waring knew how to live life to the fullest. Fishing was still important to him, and he was told that he should have oxygen before setting out. For higher altitude, he was to increase his medication. He and Ruth went fishing in March 1958 in Florida. He wrote to his office staff: "Caught a lot of fish. Am feeling fine. Thanks for peanuts and 'Snicker Snacks'!" In April 1958 he wrote to Esmond Long to say that he was sorry he could not be present when Long gave the Amberson Lecture. "I find attending medical meetings very fatiguing and must call a halt." And in answer to a question about climate put to him by his old friend: "I would rather be a live Colorado prairie dog than a dead Long Island duck." It was an oft-quoted phrase, referring to his belief in the therapeutic effects of a dry, sunny climate.

JAMES WARING served as honorary chairman of the Denver Tuberculosis Society's Christmas Seal campaign in 1958. In newspaper articles he told of the services performed by the organization—case-finding programs, tuberculin-testing projects, and a free chest x-ray program—and told the history of the Christmas Seal.[49]

In 1959 Waring was planning a fishing trip in the Virgin Islands and Florida in the winter. He wrote ahead to his cousin, Dr. T. P. (Pinck) Waring, "Would you be kind enough to set up at Susie's [Antonio's widow's] house a medium-sized tank of oxygen with flow-meter attached. I have my own hose and mask which I will bring with me." When he arrived in Savannah, he later wrote a friend, "I blew up with a severe abdominal emergency—operated on at midnight . . . had to have a dozen transfusions or so. Six weeks in the hospital." He lost his spleen, torn during surgery, and had a gall bladder "full of gallstones." In a postcard to the staff at the Webb Institute: "Greetings: Ouch! Ouch! yrs. J.J.W. P.S. More later. P.P.S. Ouch!!!"

The "preoperative diagnosis was a rupture of an aortic aneurysm," he wrote another friend, "but the operative diagnosis was a retro peritoneal hemorrhage, not from the aortic aneurysm. I had the best of medical and surgical care. . . . I seem to have survived and actually feel better right now than I have in a long time."

In previous years Dr. J. Cuthbert Owens, a vascular surgeon and a professor of surgery at the University of Colorado School of Medicine, had seen Waring as a patient for keratotic (precancerous) skin lesions, which he removed. Owens cannot recall when he first saw that Waring had a potentially life-threatening condition, but believes it was about 1954:

> He had the biggest abdominal aortic aneurysm I'd ever palpated. The surgical mortality was still too high to operate on an

> asymptomatic high-risk patient even though the first [thoracic] aneurysm was grafted by Dr. Henry Swan [of the University of Colorado School of Medicine] in 1949 and the first abdominal aneurysm was performed in Paris in 1950 by Charles Dubost. It was too early and too much of a risk to operate on anyone with the same findings electively, especially a former chairman of medicine with pulmonary insufficiency—we hadn't enough cases under our belt. But if [the aneurysm] had ruptured, we'd have to have done [the operation].
>
> Jim's lungs were awful; he was breathing oxygen—he was a "respiratory cripple." I even worried about taking off the [keratotic] lesions with a local anesthetic."

When he heard about Waring's episode in Savannah, Owens worried that he might have ruptured his abdominal aneurysm. But he had not, and they closed him up. His surgeon had an excellent reputation, and Owens breathed a sigh of relief. But in July, Waring developed shingles. To a friend he wrote that shingles was "a cruelly painful experience I assure you. I completely exhausted all my limited vocabulary of English profanity and turned on my steam in a little French, Spanish and German profanity."

For Waring, his "laboring pump" meant it was impossible for him to visit his daughter Ruth and her family when they were at their ranch in northwest Colorado. Ruth and Robert Halpenny had bought a ranch, at an altitude of 6,700 feet, in Hayden in 1959. For ten years thereafter, they and their two sons and daughter divided their time between the ranch and their orange orchards in Riverside, California. (Today the Halpenny sons have become farmers and ranchers themselves.)

After a visit with the Halpennys in Riverside, Waring wrote a friend, "Ruth is showing masterly patience in taking care of them and bringing them up." Ruth now was learning how to adapt to life on a ranch—even as a midwife for heifers. She immersed herself in 4-H activities, canned fruits and vegetables, and made dresses, an active life.

In 1959 Anne had a second son, James Waring White—who would be called Jamie—adding to James's and Ruth's happiness. Holding baby Jamie as he rocked in a rocking chair, the grandfather would say, "I'm getting my batteries charged!" The year also brought sadness when Aunt Minna died. She had been more than an aunt; she had been there in Colorado Springs when her nephew needed her, when he was taken off the train on a stretcher. She had been available when needed by others but still managed to preserve her precious independence.

That year friends made sure Waring knew how much he was appreciated. Fifty of them bought him an oil painting they knew he admired: *The Hoop Dancer,* by an Arizona painter named Ted DeGrazia. Anne remembers her father being entranced by a performance of Koshare Indian dances one year at the Warings' annual dinner for the house staff of the Department of Medicine.

Honors continued to come to Waring: Regis College in Denver honored him in 1959 with its Civis Princeps award, naming him First Citizen in the State of Colorado in Health and Welfare. Then, at the annual meeting of the Denver Tuberculosis Society on April 21, 1960, friends, colleagues, and coworkers in the field of public health surprised Waring with a "This Is Your Life" presentation. Col. James Wier, president of the society, introduced Waring's old friend, Henry Toll Sr., narrator. In a large dining room in the Albany Hotel, the assembled guests were taken on a humorous trip through Waring's life, but it was a serious tribute. Some of the narrator's words: "You urge the joint cooperation of governmental agencies, social welfare agencies, and medical agencies to aid in the improvement of the standard of living. . . . Doctor, humanitarian, peacemaker in interpreting public health needs to organized medicine, fighter against disease."

Afterward Henry Toll showed slides of old family pictures. When a slide of Waring sitting with his Halpenny grandchildren in a covered wagon was shown, the guest of honor commented: "There I am, arriving in Colorado in a covered wagon!" Ruth said a few touching words, including, "No one could have had a better life partner." Then Waring was presented with a leather volume containing 150 letters and telegrams from his friends throughout the nation; a silver paper knife from the board of directors; and a check from the Denver Tuberculosis Society to the Colorado Foundation for Research in Tuberculosis.

The death in September 1960 of J. Carroll Bell, M.D., of the Webb Institute affected Waring deeply. Bell had interned at Colorado General and had become friends with Waring during the next five years while in an internal residency program. He later worked at the Webb Institute and managed to coauthor a book on chemotherapy before his death from amyotrophic lateral sclerosis (Lou Gehrig's disease).

Waring continued to stay involved with the institute and took pleasure in showing it to friends such as Dr. Leonard Freeman, one-time head of surgery at the medical school. In November 1961 Waring gave a tour of the institute to an old friend, J. Arthur Myers, M.D., of Minneapolis. Myers later wrote of this visit: "This was a most pleasant occasion. We saw him as vivacious as ever, reminiscing and planning for future developments of the Institute. His enthusiasm in promotion of the Institute was so great that, although it was late at night, he insisted upon taking us on a tour of his inspection of the building and showing us views of planned additions. His most pleasing comment of the evening . . . was that the directorship [referring to Dr. Roger Mitchell] was in such excellent hands."

Health considerations did not diminish Waring's efforts to raise matching funds for an addition to the Webb Building. What Osler said in 1913 applied as well half a century later: "To have lived through a revolution, to have seen a new birth of science, a new dispensation of health, reorganized medical schools . . . is not given to every generation." It was a time of dramatic change, with revolutionary advances in chemotherapy and in the biological sciences, in increased funding for research, and improved facilities.

JAMES WARING had a heart murmur. His old friend and ex-student, Jack Durrance, says, "He knew he was going to die from it, and he wasn't afraid of it. . . . One time he said, 'Jack, I want you to listen to my chest.' I said, 'I don't want to listen to your chest. You have plenty of doctors; I'd just as soon not treat you, not know about you, if you don't mind.' He did mind, a little bit. He said, 'I just want you to listen.' And I never did. Nowadays he could be operated on—the valve didn't shut properly, and allowed blood to leak backward. But with his lung disease, he might not have stood it [an operation]. Hard to say."

Dr. Wallace Livingston, as a resident and as chief resident (1947–1948) at the University of Colorado School of Medicine, says he was somewhat in awe of Waring: "I always said my two best teachers in internal medicine were my father and Dr. Waring." Therefore, when he had a call to see the professor emeritus it was with trepidation that he went. Livingston explains that Waring was actually the patient of Robert Liggett, one of his partners, but it was the weekend and Liggett was off. "I remember making rounds. . . . [Our practice] rotated weekend calls. . . . [Dr. Waring] intimidated me, listening to his heart; he had aortic stenosis. [He was] revered by everyone. Gentleman and scholar, a man everyone looked up to. I fantasized about being a teacher like Dr. Waring . . . I think of Dr. Waring often."

On May 10 Waring spoke to the Thursday Lunch Club, to which Ruth belonged. A member later recalled, "It gave us such an insight into his extraordinary life and what he has done for the world—yes, the world."

In late May the Warings attended the annual Plant Auction of the

Denver Botanic Gardens, and the director of the gardens, A. C. Hildreth, later commented that Waring seemed "his usual witty self and we were encouraged by his improvement." Dr. Sidney Burwell, consultant to the dean, Harvard Medical School, and his wife had lunch with the Warings, also in late May.

Waring's youthful spirit still prevailed; he was as curious as ever. He had been trying that spring to find an article by Farley Mowat about raising owls—perhaps a young owl had been orphaned at The Farm.

He seemed to be better at the end of May. Anne and Ed White had planned a trip to Italy, and Waring told his daughter there was no reason for them not to depart as planned. Anne was worried about her father's frail appearance, but he had pulled through repeatedly in the past. Her mother also encouraged her to go. Jim Day of Colorado Springs later commented, in a letter to Ruth Waring, on "[Dr. Waring's] good humor and his fine spirits at our meeting" on May 31, the day the Whites departed.

That same day Waring wrote his old friend, J. Arthur Myers, that he would like to retire as president of the board of the Webb Institute and have Robert L. Stearns take his place. Two days later, on the evening of June 2, 1962, Waring said he was not feeling well and lay down on his bed. Ruth heard a sound and went into his bedroom. He had gone; aortic stenosis had taken its toll. James Waring was seventy-eight. Considering the prognosis of over half a century before, he had defied the statistics.

Daughter Ruth was with Robert at their ranch in Hayden, Colorado, when word reached them. Anne and Ed had just arrived in Florence for the night when they were informed. Within twenty-four hours they were able to return to Denver. As word spread, letters and telegrams of condolence began to arrive. One to Anne read: "If my family and friends remember me when I am dead with even a fraction of the affection with which his remember him, what a blessing for me, and how happy for them." Another friend wrote, "It's hard to see the great oaks come down one by one and Dr. Waring's death truly diminishes us all—even those of us who knew him in a more or less tangential way. . . . I have heard his name almost all of my life—always connected with things that were fine and honest."

Many were letters from patients' families. One said, "[We] owed our Mary's life to him. I remember he said, 'I won't let her slip through my fingers.'" A colleague, writing in the *Bulletin of University of Colorado School of Medicine,* said: "Since he would have disapproved any public display of sentimentality, we can only say that we were fortunate in knowing him. Many physicians will never see a 'last year's bird nest' [a phrase coined by Waring] in a chest x-ray without thinking of Lord Jim."

Robert Stearns delivered a memorial address at St. John's Cathedral in Denver on the fifth of June. He caught the essence of his friend, speaking of "a strong-willed man with a superior education, superb intelligence and warm human sympathy . . . scientist, humanist and witticist . . . combined wisdom and understanding . . . [and] love for his family. . . . We and [his family] are here today because we loved him. And we all and the human race are better off because he came, he saw, he understood, he fought the good fight—and he cured."

The torrent of letters continued to pour in to the family from all over the country. Franklin Hanger, president of the American College of Physicians, wrote, "I will always think of him sitting in his office [in the Webb Institute] last December, ill, weak, but aglow with keen humor and burning interests."

"To me," wrote a former resident, "he epitomized all that was great in those few physicians who have been able to combine a scholarly approach to medicine with a humility and gentleness of spirit that is seen in so few men."

His enduring legacy, beyond his renown as a physician with distinguished diagnostic and teaching skills, would be his ability to inspire his students, colleagues, family, and friends. In one friend's words, "We can truly marvel that his radiant spirit, his keen awareness, and his gentle courageous loving heart were never dimmed or daunted in his entire life—not even at the very end."

Ruth Waring bore stoically her great loss, telling Harriot Jardine, "I lived with the most wonderful man in the world for years, and I'm grateful."

"I think she must have been just the right wife," says a friend who knew James and Ruth Waring well. Although Ruth Waring's innate reserve prevented most people from coming close to her, those who did get to know her well tell of a wonderful relationship.

In any discussion of Ruth Porter Waring, her philanthropies naturally come into the conversation. Jeanne Erskine tells of all the people whom she helped, "and I'm sure never said a word about it." She stresses how private Ruth Waring has always been about her giving: "In so many quiet ways she contributed to the best in Denver and Colorado." But it was not only those pursuing a medical education whom she helped: she gave quietly, and often anonymously, to a wide spectrum of students.

Ruth Waring served for many years on the board of the Denver Symphony Orchestra (co-founded by her sister, Dora Porter Mason) and gave substantial financial support. She also gave to the Central City Opera Association, of which she remained a life trustee. The Central City Opera House gardens were of particular interest to her. She quietly gave money for faculty to make trips; gave to the Child Research Council; bought laboratory apparatus, and supplied money for equipment, drugs, and furnishings for the Department of Medicine, as well as a secretary's salary for ten years when state funds were unavailable. Some have spoken of her longtime support of students in need at the University of Colorado School of Medicine. In addition, a James Johnston Waring Memorial Scholarship Fund was established at the Johns Hopkins University School of Medicine. She also set up library funds at both schools. Her major medical contributions for many years went to the Webb-Waring Lung Institute.

In 1959 Anna Reynolds Garrey (Mrs. George) and Ruth Waring were awarded the Medals of Merit by the Garden Club of America; both were among the founders of the Garden Club of Denver. The pair also assisted in the founding of the Botanic Gardens Foundation of Denver; Ruth Waring served on its board for many years and was a lifetime member. That same year, she presented the Botanic Gardens House at 909 York Street in memory of her father, Henry M. Porter. The house, designed by Jacques Benedict, holds the administrative offices of the Botanic Gardens. Ruth Waring also gave the brick building used as a children's garden shelter; auxiliary greenhouses with adjoining laboratory rooms; and the Prairie Garden, named for her mother, Laura Smith Porter. Within the gardens' Helen Fowler Library is the Waring Book Room, which houses a precious collection of books about plants, especially those with medical properties, some dating back as far as the sixteenth and seventeenth centuries.

Until age ninety-seven Ruth Porter Waring rode several miles each day on her exercise bicycle. And until a few months after her one-hundredth birthday she continued to have lunch one day a week at the Denver Country Club with her old friend, Alice McWhinney, and grandson, James Waring White (Anne's second son). Despite diminished eyesight and hearing, with her independent spirit intact, she typically disdained being helped up the club's stairs by the solicitous doorman. Until a bad fall in 1990, she also had breakfast one morning a week with her grandson Jamie.

Atop the berm in the Wingsong Garden of Denver Botanic Gardens is a cultivar of dwarf Russian almond, Prunus tenella, given the designation "Ruth's 100th" in honor of her one hundredth birthday in 1989. Ken Slump, horticulturist in the plants collections department, writing in *The Green Thumb,* describes it as "a sturdy shrub which is adorned with hundreds of small pink flowers in early spring." Ruth Waring died in 1993 at the age of 103. To the end, she remained grateful for her years with James Waring.

ON THE RECOMMENDATION of Joel A. H. Webb and Marka Stewart—a son and a daughter of Webb—the name of the Webb Institute was changed to the Webb-Waring Institute for Medical Research. Robert Stearns succeeded James Waring as president of the board of trustees, as Waring had hoped he would. A third floor had been added to the building before James Waring's death, and the immediate goal toward which he had been working—the addition of fourth and fifth floors—was realized in 1964. Luther L. Terry, M.D., the surgeon general of the United States, spoke at the dedication of the additional floors.

Although tuberculosis still kills millions of people, primarily in Third World countries, its incidence in the United States continued to decline until the mid-1980s. At the same time, millions of Americans suffered disabling lung conditions, and respiratory deaths grew. With these escalating numbers, the focus of the institute shifted to chronic bronchitis, emphysema, asthma, and other lung diseases. In 1971, the institute's name was changed again, this time to the Webb-Waring Lung Institute.[50]

Over the years, the institute has been a leader in the study of cellular immunology. After ten years of labor, in 1969 Alfred Crowle, Ph.D., professor of microbiology and head of the Division of Immunology, announced a new tuberculosis vaccine, which he described as a "non-living antigen extracted by the action of the enzyme trypsin on killed TB bacilli." Unlike BCG, the vaccine did not cause the tuberculin test to read positive. The expensive, wide-scale testing necessary to prove its efficacy, however, was never carried out. Crowle's macrophage model of human tuberculosis enables researchers to examine all aspects of the disease at the cellular and molecular levels under laboratory conditions. Crowle and Dr. David W. Talmage, who served as director of research from 1973 to 1983, made notable discoveries in various aspects of immunology, some having to do with transplant rejection and cancer growth. Talmage also devised ways to prevent transplantation rejection by treating organs with oxygen, and Dr. Giles Filley developed and demonstrated the clinical usefulness of carbicarb, which is superior to bicarbonate, the traditional treatment of acidosis. He also is credited with devising a test for oxygen diffusion (the movement of oxygen between the air and the blood in the lung), the Filley test.

Dr. Roger Mitchell developed a leading pulmonary disease training program at the University of Colorado Health Sciences Center, which Dr. Thomas Petty enlarged and made highly effective by incorporating the care of the critically ill. Clinical training was offered at five hospitals (Colorado General, Denver General, General Rose, National Jewish, and Veterans Administration) in combination with the basic science of the Webb-Waring Institute. Petty, who served as president and scientific director of the institute from 1983 to 1989, was a pioneer in the treatment of patients with chronic obstructive pulmonary disease (COPD) with portable oxygen.

M. Laurance Morse, Ph.D., professor of biochemistry, biophysics, and genetics, has been a leader in bacterial genetics; he also has studied inheritance factors in human lung disease. Oscar K. Reiss, Ph.D., worked out the biochemistry of pulmonary surfactant, a detergent-like substance that lines the air spaces of the lung and is required for normal respiration. Albert E. Vatter, Ph.D., an expert in the use of the electron microscope and head of the Division of Cell Biology, discovered the structure of surfactant with Richard J. Sanderson, Ph.D.

A rich part of the history of the Webb-Waring Institute will come to a close with the retirement of Drs. Talmage, Reiss, Morse, Crowle, and Vatter. In the 1990s, the scientific process at Webb-Waring remains unchanged from the days of Drs. Webb and Waring; what *has* changed are the tools that assist the scientist, and the foundation of knowledge underlying the research. With the assistance of computers, powerful microscopes, and genetic manipulation, scientists can study the workings of a cell at a level unknown just a few years ago.

The lung continues as an important focus. In 1989, the National Institutes of Health (NIH) awarded a five-year $2.7-million Specialized Center Grant for Research (SCOR) to a team of University of Colorado Health Sciences Center scientists, headed by John E. Repine, M.D., to conduct research into the causes of Adult Respiratory Distress Syndrome (ARDS). Webb-Waring was one of six centers selected by the NIH in 1993 to receive a five-year $6-million grant. The program will integrate six projects spanning both basic and clinical studies of acute lung injury. Work with lung surfactants used in treating Infant Respiratory Distress Syndrome (IRDS) is in the early stages of testing. Webb-Waring scientists are seeking causes for the resurgence of tuberculosis; the disease flourishes among Acquired Immune Deficiency Syndrome (AIDS) patients, as it does among the inner-city poor, who are undernourished and living in crowded conditions. Drug-resistant strains are spread worldwide by increased travel.

Another aspect of research at Webb-Waring involves oxygen. With what has been learned about the oxidative processes in lung cells has come the recognition that the same process affects the heart, brain, kidneys, and other cells. When a cell becomes sick or injured, its ability to metabolize oxygen correctly is one of the first things to suffer, and oxygen radicals are produced in far greater numbers than normally would be produced. The body has defenses against free-radical attacks called antioxidants. Alterations in antioxidants occur in at least eighty diseases, including lung and heart diseases, cancer, diabetes, arthritis, AIDS, and Alzheimer's.

John Repine, a cell biologist who had been head of the Division of Experimental Medicine at Webb-Waring since 1979, assumed the directorship of the institute in 1989. A year later the board of trustees recruited Joe M. McCord, Ph.D., a biochemist, to head the Division of Biochemistry and Molecular Biology. McCord, a pioneer in oxygen radical research, is a co-discoverer (with Irwin Fridovich, Ph.D., in 1969) of the body's built-in antioxidant enzyme, *superoxide dismutase* ("SOD"), which stops the damaging chain reaction of toxic oxygen radicals. The team of experts are seeking clues to rapid identification of this life-threatening imbalance in order to intervene with new drug therapy to treat and prevent the many complex human diseases involving oxygen radicals.

Reflecting the broader scope of its research activities, there has been a name change—to the Webb-Waring Institute for Biomedical Research. As in years past, the institute continues to emphasize its teaching program, on three levels: college and high school students, who spend the summer in Webb-Waring's laboratories; physicians at the resident level and doctoral fellows; and postdoctoral researchers in the early phase of independent development, in training to become independent investigators. The present teaching program, under the direction and guidance of John Repine, recalls the interest, enthusiasm, and teaching skills of James Waring. The esprit de corps of the institute flourishes, with a multidisciplinary team of scientists engaged in a quest to unlock the secrets of how diseases develop. The potential for improved treatment and prevention of a wide spectrum of diseases is greater than ever before. Fac et spera! Work and hope!

Notes

AUTHOR'S NOTE: The reader will discover inconsistencies in capitalization and other matters of style between the author's text and that of quoted material from letters, books, articles appearing in journals, and newspapers. Style changes in time; for example, current usage favors lowercase with few exceptions. Preserving the style of writers of times past seemed a better goal than consistency; however, the overuse of dashes in letters–a common form of punctuation in the past–has been, for the most part, eliminated as a distraction. Some misspellings, similarly, have been changed. Generally speaking, little has been done to get between the writer of the original material quoted and the reader.

1. The reference to the yellow fever epidemic introduced his great-grandfather, Dr. William Richard Waring, whose report of the 1820 epidemic stood for years as the best on the subject.

2. Most of the facts about the family have been recorded in a family history written by J. Frederick Waring, a cousin of James W. Waring. He wrote the history in two installments, in 1940 and 1952.

3. An entry for 1835 in *Historic and Picturesque Savannah* by Adelaide Wilson notes that the Poor House and Hospital Society was incorporated upon application of William R. Waring and others.

4. Also sometimes written as 3 West Perry Street or as 3 Perry Street West.

5. A footnote in *The Houstouns of Georgia* by Edith Duncan Johnston stated that "a mourning ring engraved 'Lady Houstoun, Priscilla[,] February 26, 1775,' is owned by Miss Minna Alston Waring of Savannah. All of the present owners are lineal descendants of Sir George and Lady Houstoun." Sir George's father, Sir Patrick Houstoun, had come to this country before the Revolutionary War.

6. Yale was not alone: The Lawrence Scientific School was opened to students at Harvard in 1848.

7. A friend of James's at Hopkins was Herbert W. Evans, who later became a renowned collector of medical books. Evans's description of a famous Osler lecture is worth repeating, for James may have been present at the same lecture: "When Osler came back after his first year at Oxford

and, in the amphitheater at Baltimore, gave his famous lecture on Servetus, I was so impressed that I determined forever to take an interest in the history of medicine."

8. Saranac Lake had been "discovered" years before by such New England intellectuals as Emerson, Holmes, and Lowell, who went there to hunt.

9. In the 1850s, long before the discovery of the cause of tuberculosis, Herrmann Brehmer established a sanatorium for victims of the disease. If it was not the first, it was the earliest to survive. It was located at Gorbersdorf in the mountains of Silesia in Germany, in the middle of a pine forest. Brehmer, a botanist, had recovered from phthisis while in the Himalayas. A plentiful diet and exercise were an important part of the regimen. Soon after, another high-altitude sanatorium opened in Davos in Switzerland, offering mountain air and sunshine. Thomas Mann used the Davos sanatorium as the setting for his epic novel, *The Magic Mountain* (1924).

10. Although much of the money behind the development of the area came from the mining of gold at Cripple Creek in the hills above Colorado Springs, the main driving force behind the settlement of the city was General William J. Palmer, an entrepreneur from Pennsylvania. He completed the Kansas Pacific Railroad to Denver; next he initiated the Denver & Rio Grande Railroad. He bought a lot of land, laid out the town, and let it be known among his wealthy friends in the East that Colorado Springs was going to become the Newport of the Rockies. Easterners began to buy and build, and so many came from Great Britain that the town was nicknamed "Little London."

11. Many years before, Helen Hunt Jackson, a writer from the East, had come to live in Colorado Springs. Her concern for the plight of native Americans led her to write *A Century of Dishonor* and the popular novel *Ramona*.

12. Arriving thirty years earlier, Dr. Charles Denison wrote his impressions: "Buried in cotton-wood trees and shrubbery, with a background of hills, the city appears a refreshing change from the monotony of buffalo grass, anthills and cactus which extend north, east and south as far as the eye can reach. . . . As seen across the plains from the city, the mountains . . . present a magnificent appearance."

13. This was actually the second time the medical school had been moved to Denver. The first move was in 1893, but the University of Colorado had been taken to court by the University of Denver, which feared that the state university would raid its medical department's faculty and, with its lower fees, take away students. In 1897 the Colorado Supreme Court upheld the University of Denver's position barring the move, a ruling which lasted for thirteen years.

14. The symposium was sponsored several months after Waring's death by the Waring Society, a student association at the Univeristy of Colorado School of Medicine.

15. The class of 1908 at Johns Hopkins, which would have been Waring's original class, had only one female graduate, despite the efforts of Miss Garrett and her friends to help the cause of women in medical school. The entrance requirements of Johns Hopkins would have presented an obstacle to women, who at that time were less likely to pursue higher education.

16. In her biography of Dr. Gerald Webb, Helen Clapesattle states that James wrote Webb that when he was taken to lunch "on shad roe, asparagus, and strawberry shortcake" by Dr. Bonney, he learned that Bonney was seeking a man merely to do his laboratory work. Waring did not want to be a "lab man" but wanted to work with Bonney in all aspects of his practice.

17. In contrast, a block away was the home of Mrs. Crawford Hill, at one time the social arbiter of Denver, whose mansion had been designed in the grand classic manner.

18. According to Bernice E. Petersen in *A Jubilee History of Denver Botanic Gardens,* "This early organization urged establishment of forest reserves and asked Congress to adopt legislation to protect the forests of the public domain from destruction."

19. Benedict began his career in New York after studying in Chicago and Paris. He called his eclectic style, which incorporated features of Italian, French, and other periods, "Beaux Art" after L'École des Beaux Arts in Paris, where he had studied for several years.

20. In the 1990s, Porter Memorial Hospital, expanded to over 350 beds, has become one of the finest medical facilities in the Denver area, serving several states.

21. In recent years, Anne Waring Maer and her husband, Claude Maer, Jr., met descendants of Antonio Gogorza's brother in the Basque village of Oreja. The meeting had been arranged through correspondence. The Maers learned through an interpreter that Gogorza had returned to Oreja and bought land there before his death. Anne Maer describes the terrain as isolated, forbidding, mountainous, and rocky, and says the people live a very hard life.

22. Houstoun Waring, James's cousin, later asked him why he had said "as far as I could throw a *buffalo* by the tail," instead of the usual "bull." James said that because he was a westerner, he felt he had to give the expression a western flavor.

23. The dimensions are important to collectors. In the catalogue of the collection the dimensions are noted for a book dated 1546: "Magnificent large and complete copy almost a half inch taller and wider than the fine copy in the J. P. Morgan Library of New York City."

24. Several years later, during the war, Dr. Burnett submitted his resignation. It was accepted, and Burnett was thanked for his thirty-five years of service to the School of Medicine and its hospitals.

25. The first study of silicosis—a debilitating disease of the lungs marked by shortness of breath—was made in 1914-1915 on lead and zinc miners. A Public Health Bulletin, July 1916, stated: "Researches in pneumoconiosis and silicosis have established the fact that tuberculosis often accompanies and is a complication of these two important occupational diseases."

26. The first industrial clinic in this country was founded in 1910 at the Cornell Medical School Outpatient Department. Harvard, in 1923, began an industrial hygiene program when the School of Public Health was founded. A separate department of industrial hygiene was first established at the University of Pittsburgh in 1936.

27. The development of the full-time system can be traced to the Johns Hopkins Medical School in 1913, with financial support from the Rockefeller General Education Board. Based upon German models, the system was introduced to Hopkins by Drs. William Welch and Franklin Mall. The purpose of developing a full-time faculty was to stimulate research by taking away the need for medical professors to devote their main energies to maintaining a practice. In the ensuing years only a few medical schools received such aid. Gradually the supporters of a strict full-time plan came to see it as a compromise that would promote research and teaching more than the traditional part-time system.

28. Among Waring's papers there is no documentation of the salary situation; the Executive Faculty Minutes alone shed light on the controversy. It is, however, far too complicated to be dealt with in a few paragraphs.

29. The families were already acquainted. "His brother was my mother's pediatrician when I was a baby," Hunter says. "My mother's best friend was Susie Waring, Tono's wife. Their son, Tono Jr., was a great friend of mine until we went off to college. Susie, along with Mother, was one of that group of 'little old ladies in tennis shoes' who turned Savannah around." The group organized the Historic Savannah Foundation, which reversed the decline of Savannah's historic district. Dr. Antonio Waring also became involved in preservation work.

30. The original Gold-Headed Cane, a symbol of greatness in English medicine, was a walking stick with an engraved gold head owned by Dr. John Radcliffe, an eminent physician (1650-1714). It was the usual prac-

tice at that time for doctors to carry a cane, and the sound of its tapping as the doctor approached gave hope to many a patient, King William III among them.

31. The year 1673 signifies the year the Society of Apothecaries of London leased three and a half acres of farm land to grow plants and flowers for medicinal herbs; and 1722, the year that Sir Hans Sloane (1660-1753) saved the company from financial ruin by giving it a freehold on his property.

32. Dr. Harry Gordon came to the medical school in August 1946, the first full-time professor of pediatrics, and retroactively made Dr. Campbell a fellow in Infectious Disease in Polio, with a special grant from the Foundation for Infantile Paralysis.

33. More polio epidemics marked 1952 and 1953. Then, in 1955, came the formal approval of the Salk vaccine, followed by the Sabin vaccine. The disease lost its terror, at least in the developed world.

34. Dr. Edward Mugrage, Waring's friend and classmate, was called "Uncle Ed."

35. Other drugs had proved to be ineffective; penicillin, for example, was destroyed by an enzyme produced by the tubercle bacillus.

36. But he was not opposed to the operation under all circumstances, for he wrote, in "Seminar on Collapse Therapy and Related Treatment: Summary" (May 1951): "We can agree with Kinsella's conclusion that thoracoplasty is a time-honored and proved method of treatment for selected cases of pulmonary tuberculosis."

37. The Estes Park gathering was modeled after conferences held at Pembine, Wisconsin, where John B. Barnwell and colleagues pioneered the consecutive-case format. Dr. Durrance explains that several Veterans Administration installations around the region met at Pembine, a private club on an island near Iron Mountain, Michigan. "They let their hair down, occasionally invited a female doctor, no female help. Male audience, shouted loudly, learned a lot." He says that he and Waring had been a couple of times, and Drs. Roger Mitchell and Dumont Clark had each been a guest. All it took was for someone to say, "Let's start a Pembine type here and have it at Estes Park," and it happened.

38. Durrance's mischievous comments were not limited to "El Toro" sessions. One time he said to a resident, "If that nodule's tuberculous, I'll eat it." Later it turned out that it was, and the resident brought him a tray, covered with napkin, knife, fork and plate, with the specimen on it!

39. It has been said that Waring turned down the presidency of the American College of Physicians in order to work for the foundation. It is

true that he was offered the nomination for president-elect of that organization in 1950, but he had decided long before that he did not want more responsibilities on the national level. On March 28, 1946, he wrote Ruth from Atlantic City: "You have doubtless heard that I am first vice-president of the College. . . . I don't want anything more in the way of these responsibilities and by one or two little acts have shown the powers that be that I do not."

40. They were caught up in plans for building a new house, not far from 910 Gaylord Street, on Hawthorne Place designed by architect Burnham Hoyt.

41. Started in 1841, Brompton Hospital is on grounds that once were a part of a botanical garden founded in 1789, now surrounded by buildings. Brompton Hospital built a small sanatorium at Bournemouth in 1854, before Brehmer's—the first European sanatorium, begun in 1859—and before Trudeau in 1884.

42. In Britain, surgeons are called "Mr.," a tradition going back to the days when they were barbers.

43. A 1989 brochure from Chelsea Physic Garden tells that at the time of the founding of the garden in 1673 by the Society of Apothecaries of London, "Plants were the major source of medicines, and physicians and apothecaries were taught in physic gardens how to recognize and use them. . . . The study of plants' therapeutic properties therefore certainly lay behind the establishment of these gardens, but the plants grown in them were by no means confined to those of known medical efficacy. In time, such gardens have come to be termed 'botanic'; only Chelsea, with its strong tradition of medicinal teaching and research, has retained its original title."

44. Following his talk Waring sent biographical data about his grandfather—professor of physiology and obstetrics at that institution when it was known as Columbian College Medical Department—to John Parks, M.D., professor of obstetrics and gynecology. Parks replied that "following the stimulus which you gave us at the AOA meeting," a committee in his department was gathering information and photographs of all the past professors of obstetrics. The material would be presented in pamphlet form at a future anniversary of the department; "enlarged photographs of the former professors would be placed in the departmental lounge and library." In his own way, Waring had sparked renewed interest in a medical center's history.

45. When James had been "chasing the cure" at the Trudeau Sanitarium he found that buggy rides gave him fever.

46. The origins of his interest in the Yale collection he traced to his being mortified to find that Nathaniel Bowditch visited the Yale library in the

late nineteenth century and "found it wanting in most of the modern English, French and German scientific works he had been so long acquainted with." In 1951, when the Medical Library Association met in Denver, the Warings invited half a dozen of the officers to dinner at 910 Gaylord Street. One was Fred Kilgore, librarian of Yale Medical Library, who left for the airport carrying a big suitcase of books. The library, completed in 1941, now has one of the best historical collections in the country.

47. Dr. Frank Rogers came to Denver in 1963 to be librarian of Denison. A dedicated bibliophile, he was a strong supporter of the Waring Room. When an addition to Denison Library was built in 1977, the Waring Room had to be moved to the second floor and the wood panels put in storage when the original space became the reference reading room (indexes and abstracts).

48. The Evans Collection, donated by Ruth Waring and her sister, Dora Porter Mason, to the Denver Medical Society, needed a humidity-controlled environment. Because of the high cost of maintenance, the society decided to sell the collection at auction to help meet other expenses. The decision was very unpopular in some quarters, and an ad hoc committee was formed (with Dr. Henry Toll as chairman) to attempt to keep the collection in Denver, offering it for sums far lower than what could be obtained at auction. After several years, the committee gave up, and the books were auctioned off in New York City for $210,000. Toll salvaged several valuable unsold titles and gave them to Denison Library, including a second edition of Andreas Vesalius's *De Humani corporis fabrica* (1555).

49. Einar Holboell, a Danish postal employee, had the thought, while cancelling stamps, that if each stamp represented a small contribution toward the care of a victim of tuberculosis, much could be accomplished. The Danish government concurred, and in 1904 the first Christmas Seal was printed. Jacob Riis, a Danish journalist in the United States, publicized the idea in 1907. Emily Bissell of Wilmington, Delaware, took the idea to the American Red Cross in Washington, D.C., who took it over and ten years later turned the project over to the National Tuberculosis Association. In the intervening years the sales of Christmas Seals had raised millions of dollars for the fight against tuberculosis.

50. The need for a name change was affecting other organizations as well. In the 1970s the National Tuberculosis Association became the American Lung Association. Dr. Julius H. Comroe Jr., when receiving the 1974 Trudeau Medal, observed, "The new name implies not a specific commitment to one disease or to a group of diseases, but recognizes the lung as an essential organ with a new commitment to learn how it functions physiologically, biochemically and immunologically, how it defends itself, and how it responds to injury."

Sources

A TREASURE TROVE of family letters greatly enriched this project; the oldest, written by the subject's grandfather, dates from about 1842. Many letters written to James J. Waring from his mother survive, as do many she wrote to his brother Antonio, dating back to their school days. Similarly, many of the brothers' letters to their mother also survive, along with a few of the two brothers' letters to and from each other.

Letters to Ruth Porter from James Waring document their courtship, just as through the years of their long marriage Ruth saved his letters and telegrams. Some of her letters to Jim, along with a few of their daughters' letters to their father and mother, have also survived.

Dr. Edward L. Trudeau's letters to James Waring were valued so highly by him that a couple bear the marks of having been carried around and withdrawn to be shared with others. Correspondence from leading chest physicians of the first quarter of the century to Waring helped in constructing the chapter telling of his landmark paper on the history of pneumothorax. Letters to and from booksellers in this country and in Europe are also included in two boxes, on loan from the Colorado Historical Society, along with nine legal-sized pads containing some of Waring's research for the pneumothorax paper.

Correspondence, both professional and personal, from Waring's files maintained at what was then the Webb Lung Institute, was useful. Dr. Herbert W. Evans's letters to Waring shed light on the Warings' acquisition of the Evans collection of books.

Of particular help were two unpublished family histories by J. Frederick Waring: "Family Story for Elizabeth and Charles, 1893–1930" (1940) and "The Waring Family in Savannah; Told for Mickey Lane by his Cousin" (1952). Another profitable primary source was a thirty-one-page biography of Waring by Dr. Paul N. Anderson. Written when he was a student, Anderson quoted correspondence with many of Waring's colleagues, most of whom have since died. Another unpublished paper of value was that of Edward D. White III, a grandson of Waring: "Henry Miller Porter: Western Entrepreneur" (senior thesis, Yale University, 1980).

The Lawrenceville School, Yale University, and the Johns Hopkins

University School of Medicine provided yearbook pages for the subject as well as class rosters. Waring kept colorful scrapbooks while at Lawrenceville and Yale, showing his diverse extracurricular interests.

Waring's published papers were not all scientific; his later ones revealed much about him. His forebears were the focus of "The Family Circle," as was fishing in "The Anatomy of Angling," and his respect and strong friendship for Dr. J. Burns Amberson in "The Chest Service at Bellevue Hospital: A Better Mouse Trap." A column he wrote for *Colorado Medicine* in the 1930s, "Library Notes," gave him another forum in which to share his love of the history of medicine. Of foremost importance in documenting Waring's years at the School of Medicine were the Executive Faculty Minutes of the University of Colorado, 1924–1962. The annual reports of The Colorado Foundation for Research in Tuberculosis, later the Webb Institute for Medical Research, then the Webb-Waring Lung Institute—1924–1991—have also been invaluable. Other primary sources are: the minutes of the Denver Clinical and Pathological Society, 1917 to 1962, and the collected papers of the Waring Society, 1955–1971.

Among Waring's effects, in his home, in the Waring Room Library of the University of Colorado School of Medicine, and in his files at the Webb Lung Institute, were hundreds of clippings, often undated and publication not always identified. Local newspapers, *The Denver Post* and the *Rocky Mountain News,* provided a good deal of information about Denver and James Waring, as did the *Savannah Evening Press* about his forebears, his brother, and also James Waring.

Books, articles, and pamphlets of particular help were:

GENERAL: René and Jean Dubos, *Tuberculosis: The White Plague* (Boston: Little, Brown & Co., 1952); S. Lyle Cummins, *Tuberculosis in History: From the Seventeenth Century to Our Own Times* (Baltimore: Williams & Wilkins Co., 1949); Richard M. Burke, M.D., *An Historical Chronology of Tuberculosis* (Springfield, Ill.: Charles S. Thomas, 1938; 2d ed., 1955); Mark Caldwell, *The Last Crusade: The War on Consumption* (New York: Atheneum, 1988); Roger Mitchell, M.D., "Chest Medicine: A Brief History, in *The Oxford Companion to Medicine,* vol. 1 (New York: Oxford University Press, 1986); Arthur M. Olsen, M.D., "Historical Perspective Transition: A Personal Story," *Respiratory Times* 2 (August 1987); Robert G. Paterson, Ph.D., "Antecedents of the National Tuberculosis Association," Historical Series No. 2, National Tuberculosis Association, 1945; review by L. Fred Ayvazian, M.D., "The 55 Trudeau Medalists (1926–1980): A 75th Anniversary," *American Review of Respiratory Disease* (April 1980); Julius L. Wilson, M.S., "Five Great Teachers in the Field of Tuberculosis," *American Review of Respiratory Disease* (May 1981); Saul Benison, "Celebration of the Centenary of Robert Koch's Discovery of the Tubercle Bacillus," *Bulletin of the History of Medicine,* vol. 56 (1982).

SARANAC LAKE: Robert Taylor, *Saranac: America's Magic Mountain* (Boston: Houghton Mifflin Co., 1986); E. L. Trudeau, M.D., "A History of the Tuberculosis Work at Saranac Lake, New York," *Journal of the Outdoor Life,* May 1931; Lawrason Brown, M.D., "Trudeau's Family Tree: A Study of the Genealogy of Dr. E. L. Trudeau," *Journal of the Outdoor Life,* October/November 1934; Allen C. Krause, M.D., "Edward L. Trudeau," *Medical Pickwick,* March 1916; John A. Meyer, M.D., "Tuberculosis, the Adirondacks, and Coming of Age for Thoracic Surgery," *The Annals of Thoracic Surgery* 52 (October 1991).

JOHNS HOPKINS: Harvey Cushing, *The Life of Sir William Osler* (New York: Oxford University Press, 1940; 2d ed., 1946); Edith Gittings Reid, *The Great Physician: A Short Life of Sir William Osler* (New York: Oxford University Press, 1931); Donald Fleming, *William Henry Welch and the Rise of Modern Medicine* (Boston: Little, Brown & Co., 1954); Simon Flexner and James Thomas Flexner, *William Henry Welch and the Heroic Age of American Medicine* (New York: Viking Press, 1941); John S. Fulton, *Harvey Cushing: A Biography* (Springfield, Ill.: Charles S. Thomas, 1946); Wilburt C. Davison, M.D., "Sir William Osler: Reminiscences," *McGill Medical Journal* (April 1942); Wilburt C. Davison, "Osler's Influence," *Journal of the Association of American Medical Colleges* (May 1950); Joseph H. Pratt, M.D., "Osler at Johns Hopkins," in *Reminiscences of Osler in the Early Baltimore Days* (Baltimore: J. H. Press, 1931).

TUBERCULOSIS IN COLORADO: George B. Price, *Gaining Health in the West* (New York: B. W. Huebsch & Co., 1907); Thomas Crawford Galbreath, *Chasing the Cure in Colorado* (Denver: By the author, 1907); Isabella Bird, *A Lady's Life in the Rocky Mountains* (Norman: University of Oklahoma Press, 1879; reprint ed., 1960); C. F. Gardiner, M.D., "Early Days in Colorado," *Outdoor Life* 29 (June 1932); Charles Denison, *Rocky Mountain Health Resorts* (1880).

COLORADO SPRINGS: Helen Clapsattle, *Dr. Webb of Colorado Springs* (Boulder: Colorado Associated University Press, 1984); Marshall Sprague, *Newport in the Rockies* (Denver: Sage Books, 1961); Douglas R. McKay, *Asylum of the Gilded Pill: The Story of Cragmor Sanatorium* (Denver: Colorado Historical Society, 1983).

DENVER: Louisa Ward Arps, *Denver in Slices* (Athens, Ohio: Swallow Press, 1983); Thomas J. Noel and Barbara S. Norgren, *Denver, the City*

Beautiful (Denver: Historic Denver, Inc., 1987); Louisa Ward Arps, *Cemetery to Conservatory: A History of the Land around Denver Botanic Gardens* (Denver: Denver Botanic Gardens, 1980); Virginia McConnell Simmons, *Botanic Gardens House* (Denver: Denver Botanic Gardens, 1974); Bernice E. Petersen, *A Jubilee History of Denver Botanic Gardens* (Denver: Denver Botanic Gardens, 1980); Kris Haglund, *Denver Museum of Natural History: The First Ninety Years* (Denver: Denver Museum of Natural History, 1990); Mark S. Foster, *Henry M. Porter: Rocky Mountain Empire Builder* (Niwot, Colo.: University Press of Colorado, 1991); Ken Slump, "Waring, Honnen, Garrey: Early Supporters Commemorated at DBG," *The Green Thumb,* February 1992; Meindert Bosch, *Bridges across the Years: Ninety Years of History–The Bethesda Hospital, 1895-1985* (Bethesda PsycHealth System, 1988); Ruth Wiberg, *Rediscovering Northwest Denver* (Denver: Northwest Denver Books, 1976); Ida Libert Uchill, *Pioneers, Peddlers, and Tsadikim* (Boulder, Colorado, 1979); Charles Reyman, ed., *Porter Memorial Hospital: Sixty Years of Caring* (Denver: Porter Memorial Hospital, 1990); Ed Gallagher, ed., Porter Memorial Hospital employee orientation booklet, 1989; Henry Sewall, "Suggestions for the Administrative Control of Tuberculosis in the City and County of Denver," *Colorado Medicine* 4 (February 1907).

MEDICAL EDUCATION: Robert H. Shikes, M.D., and Henry N. Claman, M.D., *The University of Colorado School of Medicine: A Centennial History, 1883–1983* (Denver: Board of Regents of the University of Colorado, 1983); Richard W. Whitehead, M.D., and Robert L. Perkin, "Medical Education in Colorado, 1881–1971," *A Century of Colorado Medicine* ed. Harvey T. Sethman (Colorado Medical Society, 1971); Gordon Meiklejohn, M.D., and Charley Smyth, M.D., eds., *History of the Department of Medicine, 1933-1985* (University of Colorado School of Medicine, 1985); Frederick S. Allen et al., *The University of Colorado, 1876–1976: A Centennial Publication of the University of Colorado* (New York and London: Harcourt Brace Jovanovich, Inc., 1976); Abraham Flexner, *The Flexner Report on Medical Education in the U. S. and Canada* (Bulletin No. 4, 1910); "The Relation of Yale to Medicine" By William H. Welch, M.D. (*Yale Medical Journal,* November 1901); Henry Swan, M.D., ed., "Medical Education: Undergraduate Curriculum: University of Colorado School of Medicine," *University of Colorado Bulletin,* October 15, 1949; "Medical Education: Its Purpose and Its Problems," in Charles Vevier and David E. Rogers, M.D., eds., *A Current Commentary on Medical Education* (Lanham, N.Y.: University Press of America, 1987); W. Bruce Fye, M.D., "The Origin of the Full-time Faculty System" *Journal of the American Medical Asssociation,* 265 (1991): 1555-62; William Frederick

Norwood, *Medical Education in the United States before the Civil War* (New York: Arno Press and the *New York Times,* 1971).

COLORADO PHYSICIANS: Gerald B. Webb and Desmond Powell, *Henry Sewall, Physiologist and Surgeon* (Baltimore: Johns Hopkins Press, 1946); Lorenz W. Frank, M.D., "Sherman Grant Bonney," *Outdoor Life* 29 (June 1932); Elinor Bluemel, *Florence Sabin: Colorado Woman of the Century* (Boulder: University of Colorado Press, 1959); Edna Yost, "Florence Sabin," in *American Women of Science* (Philadelphia: J. B. Lippincott, 1955); James H. Baker and LeRoy R. Hafen, eds., *History of Colorado,* vol. 5 (Denver: Colorado Historical Society, 1927); Paul Nathaniel Anderson, "James J. Waring, 1883–1962: Doctor of Medicine," paper presented to the Waring Society of the University of Colorado School of Medicine, May 13, 1963, in *American Review of Respiratory Diseases* 88 (1963): 281; J. Arthur Myers, M.D., "James J. Waring," *Journal-Lancet* 84 (1964): 4–10; Thomas L. Petty, M.D., "James J. Waring," introductory notes on his contributions to the development of medical and pulmonary science, in *Rocky Mountain Medical Journal* 76 (1979): 119–24; *Dr. Webb of Colorado Springs,* cited above under Tuberculosis in Colorado.

SAVANNAH AND THE SOUTH: *1733-1933 Bicentennial Medical History* (Chatham County, Ga.: Georgia Medical Society); Adelaide Wilson, *Historic and Picturesque Savannah* (Boston: Boston Rotogravure Co., 1889); Edith Duncan Johnston, *The Houstouns of Georgia* (Athens: University of Georgia Press, 1950); James Wamsley, "Historic Savannah," *National Geographic Traveler,* May/June 1989.

INDUSTRIAL MEDICINE: Henry B. Selleck, in collaboration with Alfred H. Whittaker, M.D., *Occupational Health in America* (Detroit: Wayne State Press, 1962); Alice Hamilton, *Exploring the Dangerous Trades: The Autobiography of Alice Hamilton, M.D.* (Boston: Little, Brown & Co., 1943); Fred R. Ingram, "Division of Industrial Hygiene, University of Colorado School of Medicine and Hospitals," *Industrial Medicine* 4 (November 1945): 932-35.

PUBLIC HEALTH: Roy L. Cleere, M.D., and Rowena D. Danborn, "History of Public Health in Colorado," *A Century of Colorado Medicine,* ed. Harvey T. Sethman (Colorado Medical Society, 1971).

BOOK COLLECTING AND MEDICAL HISTORY: William MacMichael, 1827, with a foreword for the seventh edition by James J. Waring, *The Gold-Headed Cane* (Springfield, Ill.: Charles S. Thomas, 1953); William Osler, M.D., "On the Library of a Medical School," *Bulletin of the Johns Hopkins University* 18 (April 1907); Paul D. White, M.D., "Doctors and Books," *The New England Journal of Medicine,* February 24, 1938; Walter K. Frankel, M.D., "Bookplates of Famous Physicians," *The Merck Re-*

port, January 1950; T. R. Boggs, "Osler as Bibliophile," *Bulletin of Johns Hopkins Hospital* 30 (July 1919): 216; Judith Hannemann, "Four Physicians and Their Bookplates," *University of Colorado School of Medicine Quarterly,* Fall 1969; John B. Blake, "The Old and the New in Medical Libraries," address delivered in Denver, March 18, 1982, on the occasion of the gift of the rare book collection of the Denver Medical Society to the University of Colorado.

Index